RANSOM KHANYE

The Root of Health

Ginseng

Cover design by Ransom Khanye
All copyrights reserved.

No portion of this book may be reproduced in any form without written permission from the author.

ISBN:9798879558746

Also available on Amazon, about natural remedies, and by the same author:

1. **The Magic Oil: Unleashing the Power of Nature's Remedy - Castor Oil**
2. **The Magic Oil 2: More Castor Oil Miracles**
3. **Amazing Natural Remedies: Nature's Medicine Cabinet**
4. **101 Castor Oil Recipes for Health and Beauty: The Complete Guide to Castor Oil Remedies**

[Note: This book does not make claims to diagnose, treat, or cure any specific diseases or medical conditions. It is intended for informational purposes only and should not replace professional medical advice or treatment.]

FOREWORD

Welcome to the world of ginseng. In this captivating book, you'll embark on a journey through the rich history, diverse benefits, and endless possibilities of ginseng. From its humble origins in traditional medicine to its revered status as a global wellness phenomenon, ginseng has captivated the hearts and minds of generations, offering solace, vitality, and rejuvenation to all who seek its embrace.

As you turn the pages of this book, you'll discover the remarkable versatility of ginseng—from its ability to enhance energy levels and mental clarity to its profound effects on heart health, immune function, and beyond. You'll learn how ginseng's unique blend of bioactive compounds, including ginsenosides, polysaccharides, and antioxidants, work synergistically to support our bodies' innate healing mechanisms and promote optimal health from within.

But more than just a compendium of facts and figures, this book is a celebration of the human spirit and our eternal quest for vitality, resilience, and well-being. It's a testament to the power of nature to nurture, heal, and inspire us on our journey through life.

May this book be your trusted companion as you explore the boundless possibilities of ginseng for a healthier, happier you.

With warmest regards,

Ransom Khanye

Contents

1: Unveiling the Mysteries of Ginseng

I welcome you to the fascinating world of ginseng — nature's remarkable gift to humanity. In this chapter, we are going to embark on a journey to uncover the secrets of this extraordinary plant, renowned for its unparalleled health benefits and rich cultural heritage. Prepare to be captivated as we delve into the essence of ginseng, exploring its origins, significance in traditional medicine, and the tantalizing array of wonders it holds within its humble roots.

Definition of Ginseng

Let us begin by unraveling the essence of ginseng. Ginseng, derived from the Chinese term "renshen," which translates to "man root," is a perennial plant native to the cool, mountainous regions of Asia and North America. Its botanical name, Panax, derives from the Greek word "panacea," meaning "cure-all," a testament to the revered status ginseng has held in traditional medicine for millennia.

Characterized by its distinctive forked shape and fleshy, aromatic roots, ginseng belongs to the Araliaceae family, which includes other esteemed medicinal plants such as ginseng's close relatives, eleuthero (Siberian ginseng) and American ginseng. Ginseng's roots, which typically take four to six years to mature, are treasured for their potent therapeutic properties and adaptogenic qualities — the ability to help the body adapt to stress and maintain balance.

Significance of Ginseng in Traditional Medicine

For centuries, ginseng has occupied a revered position in the annals of traditional medicine, revered by healers and herbalists for its multifaceted healing abilities. In ancient China, ginseng was considered a symbol of longevity and vitality, coveted by emperors and scholars alike for its rejuvenating effects on the mind, body, and spirit.

In traditional Chinese medicine (TCM), ginseng is classified as a superior herb, esteemed for its ability to tonify qi (vital energy), nourish the spleen and lungs, and invigorate the body's innate healing capacities. It is often prescribed to address a myriad of health concerns, from fatigue and weakness to poor digestion and immune dysfunction. Similarly, indigenous peoples of North America revered ginseng as a sacred plant with potent medicinal properties, employing it as a panacea for various ailments.

Overview of the Book's Content

Now that we've laid the groundwork, let me tantalize you with a glimpse of the bountiful treasures awaiting you in the pages ahead. In this comprehensive guide to ginseng, we'll embark on an exhilarating exploration of its diverse forms, cultivation methods, and therapeutic applications. Prepare to be enlightened as we uncover the science behind ginseng's healing powers, from its rich array of bioactive compounds to its profound effects on physiological health and well-being.

But that's not all – our journey doesn't end there. We'll delve into the myriad benefits of ginseng, from its role in enhancing cognitive function and promoting cardiovascular health to its potent anti-inflammatory and immune-modulating properties. Along the way, we'll discover practical tips for incorporating ginseng into your daily life, whether through nourishing herbal teas, invigorating culinary creations, or convenient dietary supplements.

Are you ready to embark on this transformative odyssey through the realm of ginseng? Prepare to be enlightened, inspired, and empowered as we unlock the secrets of this extraordinary botanical treasure. Your journey to optimal health and vitality begins now.

Sources:
- Bensky, D., & Gamble, A. (1986). Chinese herbal medicine: Materia medica. Eastland Press.
- Duke, J. A., & Ayensu, E. S. (1985). Medicinal plants of China. Reference Publications.
- Winston, D., & Maimes, S. (2007). Adaptogens: Herbs for strength, stamina, and stress relief. Healing Arts Press.

2: Tracing the Roots of Ginseng's Legacy

From its humble beginnings in the mist-shrouded mountains of Asia to its rise as a revered global commodity, the tale of ginseng is a testament to the enduring allure of nature's treasures.

Origins of Ginseng Cultivation

Our journey begins in the verdant valleys and rugged peaks of ancient Asia, where ginseng first took root in the fertile soil of the earth. For millennia, indigenous peoples of China, Korea, and Siberia revered ginseng as a sacred plant, harvesting it from the wild with reverence and respect. Legends abound of wise sages and mystical beings who sought out ginseng's elusive presence, believing it to be the key to eternal youth and wisdom.

As demand for ginseng grew, so too did the need for sustainable cultivation methods. Enterprising farmers in China and Korea began cultivating ginseng in carefully tended gardens, mimicking the natural conditions of its wild habitat to nurture the plant to maturity. These early efforts laid the foundation for modern ginseng cultivation, transforming ginseng from a rare commodity to a thriving agricultural industry.

Historical Uses of Ginseng in Various Cultures

Across the centuries and continents, ginseng's reputation as a panacea for health and vitality spread like wildfire, captivating the imaginations of healers and herbalists from East to West. In ancient China, ginseng was revered as the "king of herbs," prized for its ability to tonify qi (vital energy), nourish the spleen and lungs, and restore balance to the body's essential functions. It was often prescribed to emperors and nobles as a symbol of longevity and prosperity.

Similarly, indigenous peoples of North America cherished ginseng as a sacred plant with potent healing properties, employing it as a remedy for various ailments, from fatigue and weakness to digestive disorders and respiratory ailments. The Cherokee, Iroquois, and other Native American tribes revered ginseng as a gift from the Great Spirit, using it in spiritual ceremonies and medicinal preparations.

Ginseng's Journey to Becoming a Global Commodity

As trade routes expanded and empires rose and fell, ginseng found its way into the hands of merchants and explorers, traversing oceans and continents to distant shores. In the 18th and 19th centuries, ginseng fever swept across Europe and North America, fueling a frenzied demand for this exotic botanical treasure. Ginseng became a coveted commodity, fetching exorbitant prices in bustling marketplaces from London to New York.

Today, ginseng continues to command global attention as a prized ingredient in traditional medicine, dietary supplements, and wellness products. Cultivation practices have evolved, with ginseng farms spanning the globe from Asia to North America, supplying the growing demand for this revered botanical treasure.

As we reflect on ginseng's remarkable journey through the annals of history, one thing becomes abundantly clear — its legacy is far from over. Join us as we delve deeper into the mysteries of ginseng's healing powers, uncovering the science behind its therapeutic effects and exploring its myriad applications for health and well-being.

Sources:
- Bown, D. (2007). The Herb Society of America New Encyclopedia of Herbs & Their Uses. Dorling Kindersley Publishing.
- Foster, S., & Johnson, R. L. (2014). National Geographic Guide to Medicinal Herbs: The World's Most Effective Healing Plants. National Geographic Society.
- Kim, Y. (2016). Korean ginseng: History and culture. Korea Ginseng Corporation.
- Kim, Y., & Kim, J. H. (2018). Ginseng, the Divine Root: The Curious History of the Plant That Captivated the World. Algonquin Books.

3: Unlocking the Diversity of Ginseng

In this chapter, we embark on an exhilarating exploration of three distinguished members of the ginseng family: Panax, American, and Siberian ginseng. Prepare to be captivated as we uncover the distinctive characteristics, geographic origins, and health benefits of each, illuminating the rich tapestry of ginseng's botanical diversity.

The Enigmatic Panax Ginseng

We begin with the undisputed king of ginseng – Panax ginseng, also known as Asian or Korean ginseng. Nestled in the lush forests and mountainous regions of East Asia, Panax ginseng has been revered for centuries for its potent medicinal properties and adaptogenic qualities. Characterized by its gnarled roots and delicate leaves, Panax ginseng is prized for its ability to enhance vitality, boost cognitive function, and promote overall well-being.

The All-American Ginseng

Next, we turn our gaze to the verdant valleys and wooded hillsides of North America, where American ginseng reigns supreme. With its smooth, elongated roots and vibrant green foliage, American ginseng offers a refreshing twist on its Asian counterpart. Revered by indigenous peoples for its cooling and calming properties, American ginseng is celebrated for its ability to support immune function, soothe digestive woes, and mitigate the effects of stress and fatigue.

The Resilient Siberian Ginseng

Last but not least, we venture into the untamed wilderness of Siberia, where Siberian ginseng thrives amidst the harsh, unforgiving terrain. Despite its name, Siberian ginseng – also known as eleuthero – is not a true ginseng but rather a distant cousin with similar adaptogenic properties. Resilient and robust, Siberian ginseng is prized for its ability to increase stamina, enhance athletic performance, and fortify the body against the ravages of stress and exhaustion.

Comparative Analysis of Health Benefits

Now that we've acquainted ourselves with each member of the ginseng family, let's delve deeper into their respective health benefits, comparing and contrasting their therapeutic effects with keen insight and discernment.

Panax ginseng, with its rich concentration of ginsenosides and bioactive compounds, is renowned for its ability to enhance cognitive function, boost energy levels, and support cardiovascular health. It is often prescribed to combat fatigue, improve memory and concentration, and promote overall vitality and longevity.

American ginseng, on the other hand, is prized for its cooling and nourishing properties, making it an ideal choice for individuals seeking to balance and harmonize their body's natural rhythms. It is revered for its ability to support immune function, soothe digestive discomfort, and mitigate the effects of stress and anxiety.

Meanwhile, Siberian ginseng – though not a true ginseng – boasts its own impressive array of health benefits, particularly in the realm of athletic performance and endurance. It is prized by athletes and fitness enthusiasts for its ability to increase stamina, improve physical performance, and accelerate recovery from intense exercise.

Embracing Diversity in Ginseng

As we draw to a close on our exploration of ginseng's diverse tapestry, one thing becomes abundantly clear – each variety of ginseng offers its own unique blend of therapeutic properties and health benefits. Whether you're seeking to enhance cognitive function, support immune health, or boost physical performance, there's a variety of ginseng to suit your needs and preferences.

As you continue on your journey through the pages of this book, I invite you to embrace the rich diversity of ginseng, allowing its multifaceted charms to enrich your life and invigorate your well-being. Your adventure into the world of ginseng has only just begun – who knows what wonders await you in the chapters ahead?

Sources:
- Duke, J. A., & Ayensu, E. S. (1985). Medicinal plants of China. Reference Publications.
- Foster, S., & Johnson, R. L. (2014). National Geographic Guide to Medicinal Herbs: The World's Most Effective Healing Plants. National Geographic Society.
- Kim, Y. (2016). Korean ginseng: History and culture. Korea Ginseng Corporation.
- Kim, Y., & Kim, J. H. (2018). Ginseng, the Divine Root: The Curious History of the Plant That Captivated the World. Algonquin Books.

4: The Mystery of Red Ginseng and White Ginseng

Let us now go through the enchanting realm of red ginseng and white ginseng, two distinguished varieties that captivate the senses and nourish the soul. Join me as we unravel the secrets of their production, explore their sensory delights, and uncover the unique health benefits and uses that set them apart.

The Transformative Journey: From Earth to Elixir

The journey of ginseng begins deep within the fertile soil of its native habitats, where tender roots push their way through the earth in search of nourishment and vitality. Harvested at the peak of their potency, these humble roots embark on a transformative journey that culminates in the creation of two distinct varieties: red ginseng and white ginseng.

For white ginseng, the process is one of simplicity and elegance. Freshly harvested roots are carefully washed and dried to preserve their natural color and flavor, resulting in a delicate, ivory-hued root with a subtle, sweet taste. This gentle processing method ensures that the essence of the ginseng plant remains intact, offering a pure and unadulterated herbal experience.

In contrast, red ginseng undergoes a more rigorous and intensive process known as steaming and drying. This transformative technique involves steaming the roots at high temperatures, which imparts a rich, reddish hue to the roots and enhances their therapeutic properties. After steaming, the roots are carefully dried, locking in their potent compounds and creating a bold and robust flavor profile that sets red ginseng apart.

A Symphony of Senses: Exploring Taste, Aroma, and Appearance

As we delve deeper into the sensory world of ginseng, let us take a moment to savor the nuances of red ginseng and white ginseng, from their captivating colors to their enticing aromas and flavors.

White ginseng, with its pale, ivory color and delicate aroma, offers a subtle and refreshing experience for the senses. Its flavor is mild and slightly sweet, with hints of earthiness that linger on the palate. Whether enjoyed as a soothing cup of tea or incorporated into culinary creations, white ginseng envelops the senses in a gentle embrace, imparting a sense of calm and vitality.

In contrast, red ginseng boasts a rich, ruby-red color and a bold, invigorating aroma that commands attention. Its flavor is robust and complex, with notes of spice and warmth that dance across the taste buds. Whether brewed into a steaming cup of tea or infused into traditional herbal remedies, red ginseng awakens the senses and invigorates the spirit, leaving a lasting impression of vitality and well-being.

Unlocking the Health Benefits and Uses

Now, let us turn our attention to the remarkable health benefits and uses of red ginseng and white ginseng, each offering its own unique blend of therapeutic properties and potential.

White ginseng, with its gentle and balancing nature, is often used to support overall well-being and promote mental clarity and focus. It is prized for its adaptogenic qualities, which help the body adapt to stress and maintain a sense of equilibrium. Additionally, white ginseng is believed to support digestive health, boost immune function, and promote healthy aging, making it a versatile and valuable ally in the quest for vitality and longevity.

On the other hand, red ginseng, with its potent and revitalizing properties, is renowned for its ability to enhance physical endurance, combat fatigue, and improve stamina and performance. It is often used by athletes and fitness enthusiasts to support peak performance and accelerate recovery from intense exercise. Additionally, red ginseng is revered for its immune-modulating properties, making it a popular choice for bolstering the body's natural defenses and promoting overall resilience and vitality.

Embracing the Diversity of Ginseng Varieties

As we conclude our exploration of red ginseng and white ginseng, let us celebrate the rich tapestry of diversity that defines the world of ginseng. Whether you prefer the delicate sweetness of white ginseng or the bold richness of red ginseng, there is a variety to suit every palate and preference. So, dear reader, as you continue on your journey through the world of ginseng, I invite you to embrace the diversity of its varieties and allow their unique qualities to enrich your life and invigorate your well-being. Your adventure into the realm of ginseng has only just begun – who knows what wonders await you in the chapters ahead?

Sources:
- Kim, Y. (2016). Korean ginseng: History and culture. Korea Ginseng Corporation.
- Kim, Y., & Kim, J. H. (2018). Ginseng, the Divine Root: The Curious History of the Plant That Captivated the World. Algonquin Books.
- Winston, D., & Maimes, S. (2007). Adaptogens: Herbs for strength, stamina, and stress relief. Healing Arts Press.

5: Treasure: The Art of Ginseng Cultivation

Step into the enchanting world of ginseng cultivation, where ancient wisdom and modern innovation converge to nurture nature's most precious treasure. In this chapter, we embark on a journey through the verdant fields and shaded forests where ginseng thrives, exploring the environmental requirements, cultivation methods, and harvesting techniques that bring this revered botanical to life. Join me as we delve into the secrets of ginseng cultivation, unlocking the mysteries of soil, sun, and sustainability along the way.

The Harmony of Nature: Environmental Requirements for Cultivating Ginseng

At the heart of ginseng cultivation lies a deep reverence for the natural world, where soil, climate, and topography intertwine to create the perfect conditions for ginseng to flourish. Ginseng thrives in cool, temperate climates with well-drained soil and ample shade, making it ideally suited to regions with rich organic matter and gentle slopes.

In terms of soil, ginseng prefers loamy, well-aerated soils with a slightly acidic pH level, typically ranging from 5.5 to 6.5. These conditions provide the optimal balance of nutrients and moisture retention, ensuring that ginseng roots develop strong and healthy.

Additionally, ginseng requires ample shade to thrive, as direct sunlight can scorch its delicate leaves and inhibit root growth. Forested areas with dappled sunlight or shaded canopies provide the ideal environment for cultivating ginseng, protecting the plants from harsh sunlight and promoting even growth.

Cultivation Methods and Best Practices: Nurturing Ginseng from Seed to Sprout

As we dive deeper into the art of ginseng cultivation, let us explore the methods and practices that guide growers in nurturing this precious botanical from seed to sprout. Ginseng cultivation typically begins with the planting of seeds or transplanting of seedlings into prepared beds, where they are carefully nurtured and tended to throughout the growing season.

One of the most common cultivation methods is known as the "wild-simulated" approach, which seeks to mimic the natural habitat of wild ginseng as closely as possible. This involves planting seeds or seedlings in shaded forested areas with minimal disturbance, allowing the plants to grow and develop at their own pace.

Another method, known as "field cultivation," involves planting ginseng in carefully cultivated beds or rows, where they receive regular care and maintenance. This approach allows for greater control over growing conditions and yields, making it a popular choice for commercial growers.

Regardless of the cultivation method employed, ginseng requires regular attention and care throughout the growing season, including watering, weeding, and pest management. By providing the necessary nutrients and protection from environmental stressors, growers can ensure that their ginseng plants thrive and reach their full potential.

Harvesting and Processing Techniques: Preserving the Essence of Ginseng

As the growing season draws to a close, the time comes to harvest the fruits of our labor and reap the rewards of a bountiful harvest. Ginseng roots are typically harvested in the fall, once they have reached maturity and developed the desired size and shape.

Harvesting ginseng requires patience and precision, as the roots must be carefully unearthed to avoid damage and preserve their therapeutic properties. Specialized tools such as digging forks or hand trowels are used to gently loosen the soil around the roots, allowing them to be lifted from the ground with minimal disturbance.

Once harvested, ginseng roots are carefully washed and dried to remove any excess soil and moisture. Depending on the desired end product, the roots may be further processed into various forms, including whole roots, sliced roots, or powdered extracts.

Throughout the harvesting and processing process, it is essential to handle ginseng roots with care and respect, ensuring that their delicate balance of nutrients and bioactive compounds remains intact. By preserving the essence of ginseng, growers can create products of exceptional quality and potency, worthy of the plant's revered status in traditional medicine.

Cultivating a Legacy of Health and Vitality

As we conclude our journey through the art of ginseng cultivation, let us pause to reflect on the profound legacy of health and vitality that this remarkable botanical has bestowed upon humanity. From its humble beginnings in the shaded forests of Asia to its global prominence as a symbol of well-being and longevity, ginseng embodies the timeless wisdom of nature and the boundless potential of human ingenuity.

So as you continue on your journey through the world of ginseng, I invite you to embrace the art of cultivation with reverence and gratitude, knowing that each seed planted and root harvested represents a precious gift from the earth. Your adventure into the realm of ginseng cultivation has only just begun – who knows what wonders await you in the fields and forests of your own backyard?

Sources:
- Foster, S., & Johnson, R. L. (2014). National Geographic Guide to Medicinal Herbs: The World's Most Effective Healing Plants. National Geographic Society.
- Kim, Y. (2016). Korean ginseng: History and culture. Korea Ginseng Corporation.
- Kim, Y., & Kim, J. H. (2018). Ginseng, the Divine Root: The Curious History of the Plant That Captivated the World. Algonquin Books

6: Science Behind Healing Properties

Welcome to the captivating world of ginseng, where ancient wisdom meets modern science in a symphony of healing. In this chapter, we delve deep into the intricate web of molecular magic that underpins ginseng's remarkable therapeutic effects. Join me as we unravel the mystery of ginseng's healing properties, exploring the fascinating world of ginsenosides, mechanisms of action, and the scientific research that validates its centuries-old reputation as nature's panacea.

The Power of Ginsenosides: Nature's Miracle Molecules

At the heart of ginseng's healing prowess lies a group of bioactive compounds known as ginsenosides, each one a tiny powerhouse of therapeutic potential. These remarkable molecules are unique to ginseng, offering a diverse array of health benefits that span the spectrum from immunity to cognition and beyond.

Ginsenosides are classified into various subtypes, including Rb1, Rg1, Re, and Rd, each with its own distinct molecular structure and biological activity. These compounds work in harmony to modulate the body's physiological processes, acting as adaptogens to help the body adapt to stress, enhance energy metabolism, and promote overall well-being.

Mechanisms of Action: Unlocking the Secrets of Ginseng's Effects

As we peer into the inner workings of the body, we uncover the myriad ways in which ginseng exerts its healing influence. From the cellular level to the systemic level, ginsenosides interact with a multitude of molecular targets, orchestrating a symphony of biochemical reactions that culminate in profound health benefits.

One key mechanism of action is ginseng's ability to modulate the body's stress response, helping to regulate the release of stress hormones such as cortisol and adrenaline. By buffering the effects of stress, ginseng helps to maintain a state of balance and equilibrium, reducing the risk of stress-related illnesses and promoting resilience in the face of adversity.

Additionally, ginseng is renowned for its antioxidant properties, which help to neutralize harmful free radicals and protect cells from oxidative damage. This antioxidant activity not only supports overall health and vitality but also plays a critical role in mitigating the effects of aging and promoting longevity.

Scientific Research: Validating Ginseng's Timeless Efficacy

As we journey through the annals of scientific literature, we encounter a wealth of evidence supporting ginseng's centuries-old reputation as a potent healer. Countless studies have demonstrated the therapeutic effects of ginseng in a wide range of health conditions, from cognitive decline to cardiovascular disease and beyond.

One notable area of research is ginseng's impact on cognitive function and memory. Multiple studies have shown that ginseng supplementation can improve cognitive performance, enhance memory retention, and protect against age-related cognitive decline. These effects are believed to be mediated by ginsenosides' ability to enhance neurotransmitter activity and promote neurogenesis in the brain.

Furthermore, ginseng has been shown to exert beneficial effects on cardiovascular health, including reducing blood pressure, improving cholesterol levels, and enhancing blood flow. These cardiovascular benefits are attributed to ginsenosides' ability to relax blood vessels, reduce inflammation, and protect against oxidative stress, thus reducing the risk of heart disease and stroke.

Bridging Tradition with Modern Science

As we conclude our exploration of the science behind ginseng's healing properties, one thing becomes abundantly clear – the ancient wisdom of traditional medicine is increasingly being validated by modern scientific research. Ginseng, with its rich history and potent therapeutic effects, serves as a shining example of nature's ability to heal and nourish the body, mind, and spirit.

So as you continue on your journey through the world of ginseng, I invite you to embrace the synergy between tradition and modernity, knowing that each scientific discovery brings us one step closer to unlocking the full potential of this remarkable botanical. Your adventure into the realm of ginseng's healing properties has only just begun – who knows what wonders await you in the chapters ahead?

Sources:
- Attele, A. S., Wu, J. A., & Yuan, C. S. (1999). Ginseng pharmacology: Multiple constituents and multiple actions. Biochemical Pharmacology, 58(11), 1685-1693.
- Lee, S. T., Chu, K., Sim, J. Y., Heo, J. H., & Kim, M. (2008). Panax ginseng enhances cognitive performance in Alzheimer disease. Alzheimer Disease & Associated Disorders, 22(3), 222-226.
- Kim, H., Park, S., Han, S. J., Kim, K. S., & Choi, C. W. (2013). Panax ginseng as an adjuvant treatment for Alzheimer's disease. Journal of Ginseng Research, 37(2), 113-119.

7: Nature's Secret: Potent Power of Ginsenosides

Welcome to the mesmerizing world of ginseng, where nature's magic unfolds in the form of ginsenosides – the true stars behind this miraculous herb's healing prowess. In this chapter, we embark on an exhilarating journey into the depths of ginsenosides, unraveling their intricate chemical structure, diverse effects on the body, and the paramount importance of standardized ginsenoside content in ginseng products. Prepare to be captivated by the hidden wonders of ginseng as we delve into the fascinating realm of these extraordinary compounds.

The Chemical Symphony: Deciphering Ginsenosides' Structure

At the core of ginseng's therapeutic potency lies a family of bioactive compounds known as ginsenosides, each possessing a unique chemical blueprint that orchestrates its remarkable effects on the body. Ginsenosides are classified as triterpene saponins, characterized by a steroidal nucleus coupled with sugar moieties that form their distinctive structure.

The chemical diversity of ginsenosides is staggering, with over 100 different variants identified in various species of ginseng. Each ginsenoside is denoted by a letter and number, such as Rb1, Rg1, Re, and Rd, signifying its specific configuration and biological activity. This molecular complexity underscores the multifaceted nature of ginseng's therapeutic effects, with different ginsenosides exerting distinct physiological actions within the body.

Exploring the Diverse Effects: Ginsenosides' Impact on the Body

As we venture deeper into the realm of ginsenosides, we uncover a treasure trove of health benefits that these miraculous compounds bestow upon the body. From bolstering immunity to enhancing cognitive function, ginsenosides play a pivotal role in promoting overall well-being and vitality.

One of the most notable effects of ginsenosides is their adaptogenic properties, which enable the body to adapt to stress and maintain homeostasis in the face of adversity. By modulating the release of stress hormones such as cortisol and adrenaline, ginsenosides help to mitigate the harmful effects of chronic stress and promote resilience in the body.

Moreover, ginsenosides have been shown to exert profound effects on cognitive function, memory, and mood. Research indicates that certain ginsenosides, such as Rb1 and Rg1, possess neuroprotective properties that enhance cognitive performance, improve memory retention, and alleviate symptoms of depression and anxiety. These effects are attributed to ginsenosides' ability to modulate neurotransmitter activity and promote neurogenesis in the brain.

Standardization Matters: Ensuring Quality and Efficacy in Ginseng Products

As we navigate the landscape of ginseng products, it becomes evident that not all supplements are created equal. The potency and efficacy of ginseng formulations are heavily influenced by the standardized ginsenoside content, which serves as a critical marker of quality and consistency.

Standardization involves quantifying the concentration of specific ginsenosides in ginseng extracts and products, typically expressed as a percentage of the total ginsenoside content. By ensuring that ginseng products contain standardized levels of key ginsenosides, manufacturers can guarantee their potency and therapeutic efficacy.

Consumers are advised to look for products that bear the seal of standardized ginsenoside content on the label, indicating that they have undergone rigorous testing and quality control to meet established standards. This ensures that consumers receive the full spectrum of ginseng's therapeutic benefits and can trust in the efficacy and safety of the product.

Harnessing the Power of Ginsenosides for Health and Vitality

As we draw the curtain on our exploration of ginsenosides, we emerge with a newfound appreciation for the remarkable potency of these extraordinary compounds. From their intricate chemical structure to their diverse effects on the body, ginsenosides epitomize nature's boundless potential to heal and rejuvenate.

As you continue your journey through the realm of ginseng, I urge you to harness the power of ginsenosides and unlock the full spectrum of benefits that this remarkable herb has to offer. With standardized ginsenoside content ensuring quality and efficacy, you can embark on a path to enhanced health, vitality, and well-being with confidence and assurance.

Sources:
- Lee, S. M., Bae, B. S., Park, H. W., Ahn, N. G., Cho, B. G., Cho, Y. L., ... & Lee, Y. M. (2000). Characterization of Korean Red Ginseng (Panax ginseng Meyer): History, preparation method, and chemical composition. Journal of Ginseng Research, 24(2), 78-86.
- Christensen, L. P. (2009). Ginsenosides chemistry, biosynthesis, analysis, and potential health effects. Advances in Food and Nutrition Research, 55, 1-99.
- Jia, L., Zhao, Y. Q., & Liang, X. J. (2017). Current evaluation of the millennium phytomedicine—Ginseng (I): etymology, pharmacognosy, phytochemistry, market and regulations. Current Medicinal Chemistry, 24(4), 293-306.

8: Ginseng's Role in Traditional Medicine

Step into the captivating realm of traditional medicine as we explore the rich tapestry of ginseng's historical significance and enduring legacy. In this chapter, we journey through time to uncover the profound influence of ginseng in traditional healing practices, from ancient Chinese medicine to indigenous healing traditions around the world. Join me as we unravel the secrets of ginseng's traditional applications, remedies, and its modern interpretations in contemporary healthcare.

Ancient Wisdom: Ginseng in Traditional Chinese Medicine (TCM) and Beyond

Ginseng has been revered as a sacred herb in traditional Chinese medicine (TCM) for thousands of years, earning the esteemed title of "king of herbs" for its unparalleled therapeutic properties. In TCM philosophy, ginseng is classified as a qi tonic, revered for its ability to replenish vital energy, balance yin and yang, and restore harmony to the body.

Ancient Chinese healers prized ginseng for its adaptogenic properties, using it to strengthen the body's resilience to stress, enhance vitality, and promote longevity. It was believed that regular consumption of ginseng could fortify the body's defenses, ward off illness, and prolong life, making it a cherished elixir among emperors, scholars, and healers alike.

Beyond China, ginseng found its way into the healing traditions of various cultures around the world, from

Korea and Japan to North America and beyond. Indigenous peoples revered ginseng as a sacred plant with profound healing powers, incorporating it into their medicinal rituals and herbal remedies for centuries.

Traditional Applications and Remedies: Harnessing the Healing Power of Ginseng

Throughout history, ginseng has been used in a myriad of traditional applications and remedies, each one a testament to its versatility and efficacy in promoting health and well-being. In traditional Chinese medicine, ginseng was often prescribed to address a wide range of health concerns, including fatigue, weakness, digestive disorders, and immune dysfunction.

One of the most famous traditional remedies involving ginseng is the preparation of ginseng root tea, a simple yet potent elixir believed to boost energy, improve cognitive function, and enhance overall vitality. To make ginseng tea, dried ginseng roots are steeped in hot water, releasing their beneficial compounds and imparting a slightly bitter, earthy flavor that is characteristic of the herb.

In addition to tea, ginseng was often incorporated into herbal formulations and decoctions, combined with other synergistic herbs to enhance its therapeutic effects and address specific health concerns. Traditional healers would carefully select and combine herbs based on their unique properties and the individual needs of each patient, creating personalized remedies tailored to restore balance and promote healing.

Modern Adaptations and Interpretations: Ginseng in Contemporary Healthcare

In modern times, ginseng continues to hold a revered place in the realm of healthcare, with its traditional wisdom being adapted and interpreted to meet the needs of today's health-conscious consumers. While ginseng is still widely used in traditional herbal medicine practices, it has also found its way into mainstream healthcare as a popular dietary supplement and functional food ingredient.

Contemporary research has shed new light on ginseng's therapeutic properties, validating many of its traditional uses and uncovering new potential applications in areas such as cognitive enhancement, immune support, and metabolic health. As a result, ginseng has become a staple ingredient in a wide range of health and wellness products, from energy drinks and dietary supplements to skincare formulations and culinary creations.

Furthermore, modern healthcare practitioners are increasingly integrating ginseng into their treatment protocols, recognizing its potential to complement conventional therapies and support overall health and well-being. Whether used as a standalone remedy or as part of a holistic treatment approach, ginseng continues to inspire awe and admiration for its remarkable healing properties.

Honoring the Legacy of Ginseng in Traditional Medicine

As we conclude our exploration of ginseng's role in traditional medicine, one thing becomes abundantly clear – the timeless wisdom of ancient healing traditions continues to resonate in the modern world. Ginseng, with its rich history and profound therapeutic properties, serves as a beacon of hope and inspiration for those seeking to restore balance, vitality, and harmony to their lives.

So, whether you are sipping on a cup of ginseng tea, incorporating ginseng into your daily routine, or exploring its myriad applications in traditional and contemporary healthcare, may you find solace, healing, and renewal in the embrace of this remarkable herb.

Sources:
- Bensky, D., & Gamble, A. (2015). Chinese herbal medicine: Materia medica. Eastland Press.
- Dharmananda, S. (2002). The nature of ginseng: Traditional use, modern research, and the question of dosage. Institute for Traditional Medicine.
- Yun, T. K. (2001). Brief introduction of Panax ginseng CA Meyer. Journal of Korean Medical Science, 16(Suppl), S3.

9: Exploring Ginseng's Nutritional Profile

Moving along within our journey into the nutritional realm, we will now seek to uncover more hidden treasures within ginseng roots. In this chapter, we delve deep into the nutritional profile of ginseng, exploring its rich array of vitamins, minerals, and bioactive compounds that contribute to its remarkable health benefits. Join me as we unravel the mysteries of ginseng's nutritional bounty and discover its potential to nourish the body, mind, and spirit.

Unveiling Nature's Treasure Trove: The Nutrient Content of Ginseng Roots

Ginseng roots are not only revered for their medicinal properties but also prized for their nutritional richness. These humble roots are packed with a plethora of essential nutrients that contribute to their renowned health-giving properties. From vitamins and minerals to powerful bioactive compounds, ginseng is a veritable treasure trove of nutrition waiting to be explored.

One of the key nutrients found in ginseng roots is carbohydrates, which serve as the primary source of energy for the body. Ginseng roots also contain a moderate amount of protein, essential for muscle growth, repair, and overall cellular function. Additionally, ginseng is low in fat, making it a nutritious choice for those seeking to maintain a healthy weight and lifestyle.

Vitamins, Minerals, and Beyond: Unlocking the Secrets of Ginseng's Nutritional Bounty

In addition to macronutrients, ginseng roots are rich in vitamins, minerals, and other bioactive compounds that play vital roles in supporting overall health and well-being. Ginseng is particularly notable for its high concentration of vitamins B1, B2, and B3, which are essential for energy metabolism, nervous system function, and cellular repair.

Ginseng roots also boast an impressive array of minerals, including potassium, calcium, iron, and magnesium, all of which are crucial for maintaining proper hydration, bone health, and muscle function. Furthermore, ginseng contains potent antioxidants such as polyphenols and flavonoids, which help to neutralize harmful free radicals and protect against oxidative stress.

Nutritional Benefits for Overall Health and Wellness

The nutritional richness of ginseng roots contributes to a wide range of health benefits that extend beyond its traditional medicinal uses. Regular consumption of ginseng as part of a balanced diet has been associated with numerous positive effects on overall health and wellness.

For instance, the vitamins and minerals found in ginseng roots play essential roles in supporting immune function, cardiovascular health, and cognitive function. Additionally, the bioactive compounds in ginseng, such as ginsenosides, have been shown to possess anti-inflammatory, antioxidant, and neuroprotective properties, further enhancing its therapeutic potential.

Furthermore, ginseng's ability to modulate stress hormones, boost energy levels, and enhance mental clarity makes it a popular choice for individuals seeking to improve their resilience to stress and promote overall vitality. Whether consumed as a dietary supplement, herbal tea, or culinary ingredient, ginseng has the power to nourish the body, mind, and spirit, supporting holistic wellness and longevity.

Embracing the Nutritional Brilliance of Ginseng

As we conclude our exploration of ginseng's nutritional profile, one thing becomes abundantly clear – nature has endowed this humble herb with an abundance of nutrients and bioactive compounds that contribute to its remarkable health-giving properties. From vitamins and minerals to powerful antioxidants and beyond, ginseng offers a treasure trove of nutrition waiting to be discovered.

I want to encourage you to embrace the nutritional brilliance of this extraordinary herb. Whether sipping on a cup of ginseng tea, incorporating ginseng into your favorite recipes, or simply enjoying the benefits of ginseng supplements, I hope you find nourishment, vitality, and well-being in the embrace of nature's bounty.

Sources:
- Park, J. D., & Rhee, D. K. (2011). Ginseng, the 'Immunity Boost': The effects of Panax ginseng on immune system. Journal of Ginseng Research, 35(4), 354-368.

- Choi, K. T. (2008). Botanical characteristics, pharmacological effects and medicinal components of Korean Panax ginseng C A Meyer. Acta Pharmacologica Sinica, 29(9), 1109-1118.
- Yuan, H. D., Kim, J. T., Kim, S. H., & Chung, S. H. (2010). Ginseng and diabetes: The evidences from in vitro, animal and human studies. Journal of Ginseng Research, 34(4), 369-374.

10: Forms of Ginseng: Fresh vs. Dried vs. Extracts

In the diverse world of ginseng forms each variation offers its own unique benefits and considerations. In this chapter, we'll explore the different forms of ginseng available in the market, ranging from fresh roots to dried slices and concentrated extracts. Join me as we delve into the advantages and disadvantages of each form, empowering you to make informed decisions when selecting the most suitable form of ginseng for your needs.

Exploring the Spectrum: An Overview of Ginseng Forms

Ginseng is available in various forms, each with its own distinct characteristics and applications. Fresh ginseng roots, harvested directly from the ground, retain their natural moisture and potency, offering a crisp texture and mild flavor. Dried ginseng roots, on the other hand, have been carefully dehydrated to preserve their shelf life and concentration of bioactive compounds. Ginseng extracts, derived from either fresh or dried roots, undergo further processing to concentrate their beneficial components into a convenient and potent form.

Weighing the Pros and Cons: Advantages and Disadvantages

Each form of ginseng comes with its own set of advantages and disadvantages, depending on factors such as convenience, potency, and personal preferences. Fresh ginseng roots are prized for their crisp texture and mild flavor, making them ideal for culinary applications such as soups, stews, and teas. However, fresh ginseng roots have a relatively short shelf life and may not be as potent as their dried or extracted counterparts.

Dried ginseng roots offer the advantage of extended shelf life and increased potency, as the dehydration process concentrates their beneficial compounds. Dried ginseng roots are versatile and convenient, allowing for easy storage and transportation without compromising their nutritional integrity. However, some individuals may find dried ginseng roots to be less palatable than fresh roots due to their denser texture and stronger flavor.

Ginseng extracts, such as powders, capsules, and tinctures, offer the ultimate convenience and potency, as they deliver a concentrated dose of ginseng's beneficial compounds in a convenient and easily digestible form. Ginseng extracts are ideal for individuals seeking maximum therapeutic benefits with minimal effort, making them popular choices for busy lifestyles. However, ginseng extracts may be more expensive than fresh or dried roots, and some individuals may prefer the sensory experience of consuming whole roots.

Making Informed Choices: Considerations for Selection

When selecting the most suitable form of ginseng, it's essential to consider your individual needs, preferences, and lifestyle factors. If you value freshness and enjoy culinary experimentation, fresh ginseng roots may be the perfect choice for you. Alternatively, if convenience and potency are top priorities, ginseng extracts offer a convenient and effective solution.

Additionally, consider factors such as budget, storage space, and intended usage when making your selection. Fresh ginseng roots may be more affordable and readily available during the harvest season, while ginseng extracts may offer long-term value and convenience for daily supplementation. Ultimately, the best form of ginseng is the one that aligns with your unique preferences and lifestyle needs.

Harnessing the Power of Ginseng in All its Forms

As we conclude our exploration of ginseng forms, one thing becomes abundantly clear – whether fresh, dried, or in extract form, ginseng offers a wealth of benefits waiting to be discovered. From culinary delights to potent supplements, ginseng adapts to meet the diverse needs and preferences of individuals seeking to enhance their health and vitality.

Again I want to encourage you to embrace the diversity of its forms and explore the myriad ways in which it can enrich your life. Whether sipping on a cup of ginseng tea, savoring the flavor of dried roots, or enjoying the convenience of ginseng extracts, I pray that you may find nourishment, vitality, and well-being in the embrace of this extraordinary herb in all its forms.

Sources:
- Kang, S., Min, H., & Ginseng, P. (2012). Ginseng, the 'Immunity Boost': The effects of Panax ginseng on immune system. Journal of Ginseng Research, 35(4), 354-368.
- Park, J. D., & Rhee, D. K. (2011). Ginseng, the 'Immunity Boost': The effects of Panax ginseng on immune system. Journal of Ginseng Research, 35(4), 354-368.
- Choi, K. T. (2008). Botanical characteristics, pharmacological effects and medicinal components of Korean Panax ginseng C A Meyer. Acta Pharmacologica Sinica, 29(9), 1109-1118.

11: Choosing the Right Ginseng Product for You

Our journey is now of informed decision-making as we navigate the vast landscape of ginseng products. In this chapter, we'll explore the essential factors to consider when purchasing ginseng, from quality indicators and certifications to tips for avoiding counterfeit or adulterated products. Join me as we empower you to make confident choices and find the perfect ginseng product to meet your needs.

Navigating the Market: Essential Factors to Consider

As you venture into the world of ginseng products, it's crucial to consider several factors to ensure you're getting the best quality and value for your investment. First and foremost, consider the form of ginseng that best suits your needs, whether it's fresh roots, dried slices, extracts, capsules, or teas. Each form offers its own unique benefits and considerations, so take the time to explore your options and choose accordingly.

Next, pay close attention to the ginseng's origin and growing conditions. Ginseng cultivated in regions known for their pristine environments and optimal growing conditions, such as Korea, China, and North America, is likely to be of higher quality and potency. Additionally, look for products that are ethically sourced and sustainably harvested to ensure environmental responsibility and support local communities.

Quality Indicators and Certifications: What to Look For

When purchasing ginseng products, it's essential to look for quality indicators and certifications that guarantee the product's authenticity and purity. One of the most reliable certifications to look for is the Good Manufacturing Practices (GMP) certification, which ensures that the product has been manufactured according to rigorous quality standards and practices.

Furthermore, seek out products that have been tested and certified by reputable third-party organizations, such as the United States Pharmacopeia (USP) or ConsumerLab.com. These certifications verify that the product meets stringent quality and purity standards and is free from contaminants or adulterants.

Tips for Avoiding Counterfeit or Adulterated Ginseng

In a market flooded with ginseng products of varying quality and authenticity, it's essential to be vigilant and discerning to avoid counterfeit or adulterated products. One way to safeguard against counterfeit ginseng is to purchase from reputable and trusted sources, such as established herbal shops, pharmacies, or certified online retailers.

Additionally, carefully examine the product packaging and labeling for signs of authenticity, including proper spelling, grammatical errors, and official seals or certifications. Avoid products with vague or misleading claims, unrealistic promises, or unusually low prices, as these may be indicators of counterfeit or adulterated ginseng.

Finally, consider consulting with a qualified healthcare professional or herbalist for personalized guidance and recommendations based on your individual health needs and goals. They can provide valuable insights and help you navigate the complex landscape of ginseng products, ensuring you find the right product for you.

Empowering Your Journey with Ginseng

As we conclude our exploration of choosing the right ginseng product, one thing becomes abundantly clear – by arming yourself with knowledge and discernment, you can navigate the market with confidence and find the perfect ginseng product to support your health and well-being.

I encourage you therefore to empower yourself with the information and resources needed to make informed choices. Whether seeking a potent herbal supplement, a soothing tea, or a culinary delight, may you find nourishment, vitality, and joy in the embrace of this extraordinary herb.

Sources:

- Smith, T., & Kawa, K. (2019). Herbal Supplement Sales in US Increased by 9.4% in 2018, Topping $9 Billion. HerbalGram, 123, 62-71.
- Bent, S., & Ko, R. (2004). Commonly used herbal medicines in the United States: A review. American Journal of Medicine, 116(7), 478-485.
- Gafner, S., Lee, S. K., Cuvelier, M. E., & Rapisarda, P. (2017). Pharmacovigilance of herbal medicines. In A. Doucette & P. R. Blumenthal (Eds.), Botanical safety handbook (2nd ed., pp. 41-56). CRC Press.

12: Dosage Guidelines for Ginseng Consumption

Understanding dosage guidelines is key to unlocking the full potential of ginseng. In this chapter, we'll navigate the intricate landscape of ginseng dosing, exploring recommended dosages, factors influencing individual requirements, and essential precautions for safe and effective use. Join me as we embark on a journey of informed decision-making, empowering you to harness the therapeutic benefits of ginseng while minimizing potential risks.

Navigating Dosage Recommendations

Determining the appropriate dosage of ginseng requires careful consideration of various factors, including the form of ginseng, individual characteristics, and health goals. Generally, recommended dosages for ginseng range from 200 milligrams to 2 grams per day, depending on factors such as potency and concentration.

- Fresh Ginseng Roots: Typically consumed raw or brewed into tea, fresh ginseng roots may be taken at dosages ranging from 1 to 3 grams per day.
- Dried Ginseng Roots: With higher potency due to dehydration, dosages for dried ginseng roots may range from 500 milligrams to 1 gram per day.
- Ginseng Extracts: Offering concentrated doses of ginseng's active compounds, extracts such as capsules or tinctures may require lower dosages, typically ranging from 200 to 500 milligrams per day.

Factors Influencing Individual Dosage Requirements

Individual dosage requirements for ginseng are influenced by a multitude of factors, including age, weight, health status, and specific health goals. Children, elderly individuals, and those with underlying health conditions may require lower dosages or closer supervision to ensure safe and effective use.

Additionally, consider your specific health goals when determining the appropriate dosage of ginseng. Lower dosages may suffice for general health maintenance, while higher dosages may be warranted for therapeutic purposes or addressing specific health concerns. Consulting with a healthcare professional or herbalist can provide personalized guidance tailored to your individual needs.

Understanding Potential Side Effects and Precautions

While ginseng is generally safe for most people when used as directed, it's essential to be aware of potential side effects and precautions associated with its consumption. Common side effects may include insomnia, nervousness, digestive upset, and headaches, particularly with excessive dosages or prolonged use.

Individuals with certain medical conditions, such as diabetes, high blood pressure, or autoimmune disorders, should exercise caution when using ginseng, as it may interact with medications or exacerbate underlying health conditions. Pregnant and breastfeeding women should avoid ginseng due to potential risks to fetal development and newborn health.

Navigating the Path to Safe and Effective Ginseng Consumption

As we conclude our exploration of dosage guidelines for ginseng consumption, remember that knowledge, caution, and respect are your allies on this journey. By understanding recommended dosages, considering individual factors, and heeding precautions, you can incorporate ginseng into your wellness routine safely and effectively.

As you navigate the path to optimal health with ginseng, may you tread with mindfulness and responsibility. With informed decision-making and a commitment to self-care, may ginseng become a valued ally in your quest for vitality and well-being.

Sources:
- Kennedy, D. O., & Scholey, A. B. (2003). Ginseng: potential for the enhancement of cognitive performance and mood. Pharmacology Biochemistry and Behavior, 75(3), 687-700.
- Lee, J. G., Lee, Y. J., Kim, C. J., An, W. G., & Cho, J. H. (2016). Korean Red Ginseng for Functional Constipation: Clinical Evidence and Pharmacological Mechanisms. Journal of Ginseng Research, 40(4), 304-309.
- Vogler, B. K., & Pittler, M. H. (1999). The efficacy of ginseng. A systematic review of randomised clinical trials. European Journal of Clinical Pharmacology, 55(8), 567-575.

13: Brewing Ginseng Tea: Tips and Techniques

Prepare to embark on a sensory journey as we explore the art of brewing ginseng tea. In this chapter, we'll dive into the step-by-step process of preparing ginseng tea, uncovering variations in brewing methods and flavor profiles, and discovering tips for enhancing taste while maximizing health benefits. Join me as we unravel the secrets of this ancient elixir and unlock its full potential as a soothing beverage and herbal remedy.

The Art of Brewing Ginseng Tea: A Step-by-Step Guide

1. Selecting Quality Ginseng: Begin by choosing high-quality ginseng roots or tea bags from a reputable source. Look for roots that are firm, aromatic, and free from mold or discoloration.

2. Preparing the Water: Bring filtered water to a boil in a kettle or pot. For optimal flavor, use fresh, cold water rather than water that has been previously boiled.

3. Adding Ginseng: Place the desired amount of ginseng roots or tea bags into a teapot or mug. Use approximately 1 to 3 grams of ginseng roots per cup of water, or follow the instructions on the tea packaging for tea bags.

4. Pouring Water: Once the water reaches a rolling boil, carefully pour it over the ginseng roots or tea bags in the teapot or mug. Allow the ginseng to steep for 5 to 10 minutes, depending on your desired strength.

5. Straining and Serving: After steeping, strain the ginseng tea to remove any solid particles or tea bags. Pour the brewed tea into cups or mugs and serve hot. Optionally, sweeten with honey or add a splash of lemon juice for added flavor.

Exploring Variations in Brewing Methods and Flavor Profiles

Ginseng tea can be brewed using various methods, each offering unique flavor profiles and health benefits. Traditional methods involve simmering ginseng roots in water over low heat for an extended period to extract their essence fully. Alternatively, ginseng tea bags offer convenience and consistency, allowing for quick and easy preparation without sacrificing quality.

Flavor profiles may vary depending on factors such as the type of ginseng used, brewing time, and additional ingredients. Korean red ginseng, for example, is known for its robust flavor and slightly sweet undertones, while American ginseng offers a milder taste with subtle bitterness. Experiment with different brewing methods and ginseng varieties to discover your preferred flavor profile.

Tips for Enhancing Taste and Maximizing Health Benefits

To enhance the taste of ginseng tea and maximize its health benefits, consider the following tips:

- Add Flavorful Ingredients: Enhance the flavor of ginseng tea by adding aromatic ingredients such as ginger, cinnamon, or licorice root. These complementary flavors can help balance the earthy taste of ginseng and create a more complex and enjoyable drinking experience.

- Optimize Brewing Time: Adjust the brewing time to suit your taste preferences and desired strength. Steeping ginseng tea for longer periods will result in a stronger, more robust flavor, while shorter steeping times will yield a milder infusion.

- Sweeten Naturally: Instead of using refined sugar, sweeten your ginseng tea with natural sweeteners such as honey, maple syrup, or stevia. These alternatives add sweetness without the negative effects of processed sugars and can enhance the overall taste and enjoyment of your tea.

Embracing the Art of Ginseng Tea Brewing

As we conclude our exploration of brewing ginseng tea, may you embark on your brewing journey with confidence and curiosity. Whether steeping ginseng roots in a traditional pot or enjoying the convenience of tea bags, may you savor each sip and reap the abundant health benefits that ginseng tea has to offer.

So, dear reader, as you immerse yourself in the art of ginseng tea brewing, may you find joy, comfort, and vitality in every cup. With each brew, may you nourish your body, soothe your soul, and embrace the ancient wisdom of this revered herbal elixir.

Sources:

- Kim, Y. S., Woo, J. Y., Han, C. K., Chang, I. M., & Kim, S. Y. (2007). Radix ginseng protects against immobilization stress-induced changes in behavior and biochemical markers in rats. Journal of Pharmacological Sciences, 105(1), 94-102.
- Li, X., Liu, Y., Wang, L., Cui, S., & Li, C. (2017). Effect of ginseng polysaccharide on the urinary excretion of type 2 diabetic rats studied by liquid chromatography-mass spectrometry. Journal of Ginseng Research, 41(4), 493-498.
- Kim, H. G., Yoo, S. R., Park, H. J., Lee, N. H., Shin, J. W., Sathyanath, R., ... & Son, C. G. (2013). Antioxidant effects of Panax ginseng C.A. Meyer in healthy subjects: a randomized, placebo-controlled clinical trial. Food and Chemical Toxicology, 62, 215-221.

14: Incorporating Ginseng in Culinary Creations

Prepare to embark on a culinary adventure as we explore the versatile world of ginseng in the kitchen. In this chapter, we'll discover the culinary uses of ginseng in various cuisines, unveil creative recipes featuring ginseng as a star ingredient, and uncover cooking techniques to preserve its nutritional value. Join me as we infuse your culinary repertoire with the nourishing essence of this extraordinary herb, elevating your dishes to new heights of flavor and vitality.

Unveiling the Culinary Uses of Ginseng

Ginseng's unique flavor profile and nutritional benefits make it a prized ingredient in culinary traditions around the world. From soups and stews to teas and desserts, ginseng lends its distinctive earthy and slightly bitter taste to a wide range of dishes. In Korean cuisine, ginseng is often simmered in soups and broths to create hearty and nourishing meals, while Chinese cuisine incorporates ginseng into stir-fries, braised dishes, and herbal tonics. In Western cuisines, ginseng is gaining popularity as a versatile ingredient in everything from smoothies and salads to sauces and marinades.

Creative Recipes Featuring Ginseng

Let your culinary creativity soar as we explore innovative recipes featuring ginseng as a key ingredient. Whether you're craving a comforting bowl of ginseng chicken soup, a refreshing ginseng green tea smoothie, or a decadent ginseng-infused chocolate truffle, there's no limit to the delicious dishes you can create with ginseng. Experiment with different flavor pairings and cooking techniques to showcase ginseng's versatility and adaptability in a variety of culinary contexts.

Recipe: Ginseng Chicken Soup

Ingredients:
- 1 whole chicken, cut into pieces
- 4-5 slices of fresh ginseng root
- 1 onion, chopped
- 3 cloves garlic, minced
- 2 carrots, sliced
- 2 celery stalks, chopped
- 8 cups chicken broth
- Salt and pepper to taste
- Fresh parsley for garnish

Instructions:
1. In a large pot, heat olive oil over medium heat. Add chopped onion and minced garlic, and sauté until fragrant.
2. Add chicken pieces to the pot and cook until browned on all sides.
3. Add sliced ginseng root, carrots, celery, and chicken broth to the pot. Bring to a boil, then reduce heat and simmer for 1-2 hours, until chicken is cooked through and flavors have melded.
4. Season with salt and pepper to taste.
5. Serve hot, garnished with fresh parsley.

Cooking Techniques to Preserve Ginseng's Nutritional Value

To preserve ginseng's nutritional value and maximize its health benefits when cooking, consider the following techniques:

- Gentle Cooking Methods: Opt for gentle cooking methods such as steaming, simmering, or poaching to minimize nutrient loss and preserve ginseng's delicate flavor and aroma.
- Minimal Processing: Avoid excessive processing or prolonged cooking times, as these can degrade ginseng's active compounds and diminish its nutritional potency.
- Pairing with Complementary Ingredients: Combine ginseng with ingredients rich in vitamins, minerals, and antioxidants to enhance its nutritional value and create balanced and nourishing meals.

Elevating Your Culinary Creations with Ginseng

As we conclude our exploration of incorporating ginseng in culinary creations, may you be inspired to infuse your dishes with the nourishing essence of this remarkable herb. Whether simmering in a comforting soup, blending into a revitalizing smoothie, or gracing a decadent dessert, ginseng has the power to elevate your culinary creations to new heights of flavor, vitality, and wellness.

So, dear reader, as you embark on your culinary journey with ginseng, may you savor each moment and delight in the abundance of flavors, textures, and aromas that await. With ginseng as your culinary muse, may your kitchen become a sanctuary of creativity, nourishment, and joy.

Sources:
- Hwang, J. W., Baek, Y. M., Yoon, S., & Kim, H. Y. (2016). Ginseng-containing cosmetics. Journal of Ginseng Research, 40(4), 277-286.
- Xie, J. T., Mehendale, S. R., Wang, A., Han, A. H., Wu, J. A., Osinski, J., ... & Yuan, C. S. (2008). American ginseng leaf: ginsenoside analysis and hypoglycemic activity. Pharmacological Research, 58(1), 33-38.
- Liao, B., Newmark, H., & Zhou, R. (2001). Neuroprotective effects of ginseng total saponin and ginsenosides Rb1 and Rg1 on spinal cord neurons in vitro. Experimental Neurology, 173(2), 224-234.

15: Tinctures and Extracts: How to Use Them

Get ready to unlock the potency of ginseng in its concentrated forms as we explore the world of ginseng tinctures and extracts. In this chapter, we'll provide an overview of tinctures, extracts, and other concentrated ginseng products, offering instructions for proper dosage and administration. Join me as we delve into the applications of ginseng tinctures and extracts in herbal medicine and supplementation, empowering you to harness their therapeutic benefits effectively and efficiently.

Understanding Tinctures, Extracts, and Concentrated Ginseng Products

Ginseng tinctures, extracts, and concentrated products are potent formulations derived from ginseng roots, designed to deliver high concentrations of ginsenosides and other active compounds. Tinctures are typically alcohol-based preparations, while extracts may be alcohol-based, water-based, or produced using other solvents. These concentrated ginseng products offer convenient and versatile ways to incorporate ginseng into your wellness routine, providing potent doses of ginseng's therapeutic compounds in a concentrated form.

Instructions for Proper Dosage and Administration

When using ginseng tinctures, extracts, or concentrated products, it's essential to follow proper dosage and administration guidelines to ensure safe and effective use. Dosages may vary depending on factors such as the concentration of the product, the individual's health status, and specific health goals. Always refer to the manufacturer's instructions and consult with a qualified healthcare professional or herbalist for personalized guidance.

Guidelines for Dosage and Administration:

1. Start Low, Go Slow: Begin with a low dosage and gradually increase as needed, paying attention to your body's response and any potential side effects.
2. Read Labels Carefully: Thoroughly review the product label for information on dosage recommendations, concentration, and administration instructions.
3. Dilute as Needed: Ginseng tinctures and extracts can be diluted in water or juice to adjust the dosage and minimize potential side effects, such as gastrointestinal upset.
4. Monitor Effects: Pay attention to how your body responds to the ginseng tincture or extract, noting any changes in energy levels, mood, or overall well-being.
5. Seek Professional Guidance: If you have any underlying health conditions or are taking medications, consult with a healthcare professional before using ginseng tinctures or extracts to avoid potential interactions or adverse effects.

Applications in Herbal Medicine and Supplementation

Ginseng tinctures, extracts, and concentrated products have a wide range of applications in herbal medicine and supplementation, offering targeted support for various health concerns. Whether you're looking to boost energy levels, support cognitive function, or enhance immune function, ginseng tinctures and extracts can be valuable allies in your wellness journey.

Common Applications Include:

- Energy and Vitality: Ginseng tinctures and extracts are renowned for their energizing properties, making them popular choices for combating fatigue and promoting vitality.
- Cognitive Function: Ginseng is revered for its ability to support cognitive function and mental clarity, making it a valuable supplement for enhancing focus, memory, and overall brain health.
- Immune Support: With its immune-modulating effects, ginseng tinctures and extracts can help strengthen the body's defenses and support overall immune function, especially during times of stress or illness.

Harnessing the Power of Ginseng Tinctures and Extracts

As we conclude our exploration of ginseng tinctures and extracts, may you feel empowered to incorporate these potent formulations into your wellness routine with confidence and intention. By following proper dosage and administration guidelines and leveraging their therapeutic properties, may you unlock the full potential of ginseng tinctures and extracts to support your health and vitality. With each dose, may you nourish your body, invigorate your mind, and elevate your spirit, one drop at a time.

Sources:
- Jia, L., Zhao, Y., & Liang, X. J. (2009). Current evaluation of the millennium phytomedicine—ginseng (II): Collected chemical entities, modern pharmacology, and clinical applications emanated from traditional Chinese medicine. Current Medicinal Chemistry, 16(22), 2924-2942.
- Kim, H. G., Yoo, S. R., Park, H. J., Lee, N. H., Shin, J. W., Sathyanath, R., ... & Son, C. G. (2013). Antioxidant effects of Panax ginseng C.A. Meyer in healthy subjects: a randomized, placebo-controlled clinical trial. Food and Chemical Toxicology, 62, 215-221.
- Lee, N. H., Yoo, S. R., Kim, H. G., Cho, J. H., & Son, C. G. (2012). Safety and efficacy of Panax ginseng berry extract on serum glucose levels and lipid profiles in subjects with non-insulin-dependent diabetes mellitus. Journal of Alternative and Complementary Medicine, 18(12), 1199-1205.

16: Capsules & Tablets: Convenience vs. Effectiveness

In this chapter, we'll delve into the realm of ginseng capsules and tablets, exploring the balance between convenience and effectiveness in these popular forms of ginseng supplementation. We'll examine the advantages and limitations of ginseng capsules and tablets, explore factors that affect absorption and bioavailability, and compare these delivery methods with other forms of ginseng supplementation. Join me as we unravel the nuances of ginseng encapsulation and tabletization, empowering you to make informed choices for your health and wellness journey.

Understanding Ginseng Capsules and Tablets

Ginseng capsules and tablets offer a convenient and portable way to incorporate ginseng into your daily routine, providing standardized doses of ginseng's active compounds in a convenient, easy-to-swallow form. These formulations are typically produced using dried ginseng root powder or concentrated ginseng extracts, encapsulated or compressed into individual doses for oral consumption.

Advantages of Capsules and Tablets:

- Convenience: Capsules and tablets are convenient for on-the-go use, allowing for easy administration without the need for measuring or preparation.
- Standardized Dosing: Capsules and tablets provide standardized doses of ginseng, ensuring consistency in potency and efficacy from dose to dose.

- Long Shelf Life: Capsules and tablets have a longer shelf life compared to liquid formulations, making them suitable for storage and travel.

Limitations of Capsules and Tablets:

- Absorption Rate: Capsules and tablets may have slower absorption rates compared to liquid formulations, potentially delaying the onset of therapeutic effects.
- Digestive Factors: Factors such as stomach acidity and digestive health can affect the absorption and bioavailability of ginseng compounds from capsules and tablets.
- Potential Additives: Some capsules and tablets may contain fillers, binders, or other additives that could affect absorption or cause adverse reactions in sensitive individuals.

Factors Affecting Absorption and Bioavailability

Several factors can influence the absorption and bioavailability of ginseng compounds from capsules and tablets, including:

- Ginsenoside Content: The concentration and composition of ginsenosides in the formulation can affect absorption rates and therapeutic efficacy.
- Formulation Design: Factors such as particle size, coating, and excipients used in capsule or tablet formulations can influence dissolution and absorption rates.
- Individual Physiology: Variations in stomach acidity, gastrointestinal motility, and enzyme activity can affect

the absorption and metabolism of ginseng compounds in the body.

Comparisons with Other Delivery Methods

When considering ginseng supplementation, it's essential to weigh the pros and cons of capsules and tablets against other delivery methods, such as liquid extracts, teas, and topical preparations. Each delivery method offers unique advantages and considerations based on factors such as convenience, absorption rates, and personal preference.

Liquid Extracts:

- Advantages: Liquid extracts offer rapid absorption and customizable dosing, making them suitable for individuals seeking fast-acting effects or those with digestive issues.
- Considerations: Liquid extracts may have a shorter shelf life and require refrigeration to maintain stability and potency.

Teas and Infusions:

- Advantages: Ginseng teas and infusions provide a soothing and traditional way to consume ginseng, offering hydration along with therapeutic benefits.
- Considerations: Teas may have variable potency depending on brewing methods and quality of ingredients, and they may not be suitable for individuals sensitive to caffeine or other tea components.

Topical Preparations:

- Advantages: Topical ginseng preparations, such as creams or ointments, offer targeted delivery for localized benefits, such as skin health or pain relief.
- Considerations: Topical preparations may have limited systemic absorption and may not provide the same comprehensive benefits as oral supplementation for systemic health support.

Balancing Convenience and Effectiveness

As we conclude our exploration of ginseng capsules and tablets, may you find clarity in navigating the balance between convenience and effectiveness in ginseng supplementation. Whether opting for capsules, tablets, liquid extracts, teas, or topical preparations, may you choose the delivery method that aligns with your lifestyle, preferences, and health goals.

I hope that you may find empowerment in making informed choices that support your health and well-being as you embark on your journey with ginseng supplementation. With each dose, embrace the transformative power of ginseng, enhancing vitality, resilience, and vitality in every aspect of your life.

Sources:
- Attele, A. S., Wu, J. A., & Yuan, C. S. (1999). Ginseng pharmacology: Multiple constituents and multiple actions. Biochemical Pharmacology, 58(11), 1685-1693.
- Yuan, C. S., Wang, C. Z., & Wicks, S. M. (2002). Qi as the basis for the development of pharmaceuticals from

ginseng. Alternative and Complementary Therapies, 8(5), 518-526.

- Choi, K. T. (2008). Botanical characteristics, pharmacological effects and medicinal components of Korean Panax ginseng C A Meyer. Acta Pharmacologica Sinica, 29(9), 1109-1118.

17: Skincare: Rejuvenate Your Skin Naturally

In this chapter, we'll explore the remarkable benefits of incorporating ginseng into your skincare routine. From its ability to enhance skin health and appearance to its potential to rejuvenate and revitalize tired, dull complexions, ginseng is a versatile ally in the quest for radiant, youthful skin. Join me as we delve into the benefits of ginseng for skincare, discover DIY skincare recipes using ginseng extracts or powders, and explore commercial skincare products containing ginseng extracts.

Harnessing the Benefits of Ginseng for Skin Health

Ginseng has long been revered for its potent antioxidant, anti-inflammatory, and anti-aging properties, making it a valuable ingredient in skincare formulations. From promoting collagen production to improving skin elasticity and texture, ginseng offers a myriad of benefits for overall skin health and appearance.

Key Benefits of Ginseng for Skin:

- Anti-Aging: Ginseng contains compounds that help combat oxidative stress and free radical damage, reducing the signs of aging such as fine lines, wrinkles, and sagging skin.
- Brightening: Ginseng's revitalizing properties help promote cell turnover and skin renewal, leading to a brighter, more radiant complexion.

- Hydration: Ginseng is known for its ability to improve skin hydration levels, leaving skin soft, supple, and moisturized.
- Firming: Ginseng helps improve skin elasticity and firmness, resulting in a more lifted and toned appearance.
- Calming: Ginseng's anti-inflammatory properties can help soothe and calm irritated or sensitive skin, reducing redness and inflammation.

DIY Skincare Recipes Using Ginseng Extracts or Powders

Elevate your skincare routine with these DIY recipes featuring ginseng extracts or powders, allowing you to harness the power of ginseng in its purest form. Whether you're looking to create a revitalizing face mask, an invigorating toner, or a nourishing serum, these recipes offer natural and effective solutions for achieving radiant, healthy-looking skin.

Revitalizing Ginseng Face Mask:

Ingredients:
- 1 tablespoon ginseng powder
- 1 tablespoon honey
- 1 teaspoon yogurt
- 1 teaspoon lemon juice

Instructions:
1. In a small bowl, combine ginseng powder, honey, yogurt, and lemon juice.
2. Mix well until a smooth paste forms.
3. Apply the mask to clean, dry skin, avoiding the eye area.

4. Leave on for 15-20 minutes, then rinse off with lukewarm water.
5. Follow with your favorite moisturizer.

Commercial Skincare Products Containing Ginseng Extracts

In addition to DIY skincare recipes, you can also explore commercial skincare products containing ginseng extracts for added convenience and efficacy. From serums and creams to masks and toners, there are numerous skincare formulations on the market that feature ginseng as a key ingredient.

Key Considerations When Choosing Skincare Products:

- Ingredients: Look for products that contain high-quality ginseng extracts or powders, ideally listed near the top of the ingredient list for maximum potency.
- Formulation: Consider your skin type and concerns when selecting skincare products, opting for formulations that address your specific needs, whether it's anti-aging, brightening, or hydration.
- Reviews and Recommendations: Research product reviews and seek recommendations from trusted sources to ensure the effectiveness and safety of the skincare products you choose.

Embracing the Power of Ginseng for Beautiful Skin

As we conclude our exploration of ginseng in skincare, may you feel inspired to incorporate this remarkable herb into your daily beauty routine. Whether you prefer DIY skincare recipes or commercial products, may you experience the transformative benefits of ginseng for radiant, youthful-looking skin.

As you embark on your journey to rejuvenate your skin naturally with ginseng, embrace the power of nature to nurture and revitalize your complexion. With each application, may you feel more confident, radiant, and beautiful, inside and out.

Sources:
- Lee, H. J., Lee, Y. H., Park, S. K., & Kang, M. H. (2013). Effect of Korean red ginseng on skin enhancement. Food Science and Biotechnology, 22(1), 197-202.
- Yoon, S. L., Cha, D. S., Choi, Y. H., Kim, Y. S., & Choi, C. W. (2019). Antioxidant activity and protective effects of red ginseng extract against ultraviolet-B-induced photoaging in human dermal fibroblasts. Journal of Ginseng Research, 43(3), 411-419.
- Kim, S., Kim, M., & Kang, M. (2017). Effects of ginseng total saponin on skin barrier recovery after UVB-induced photodamage in hairless mice. Journal of Ginseng Research, 41(4), 522-527.

18: Ginseng for Mental Clarity and Focus

In this chapter, we'll dive into the fascinating world of ginseng and its profound effects on mental clarity and focus. We'll explore the compelling evidence supporting ginseng's cognitive-enhancing properties, dissect the intricate mechanisms of action on brain function and neurotransmitters, and provide practical tips for seamlessly incorporating ginseng into your daily routines to unlock enhanced mental clarity and focus.

Unveiling the Evidence: Ginseng's Cognitive-Enhancing Effects

Ginseng has garnered significant attention for its potential to enhance cognitive function and promote mental clarity. Numerous studies have provided compelling evidence supporting ginseng's cognitive-enhancing effects, highlighting its ability to improve memory, concentration, and overall cognitive performance.

Key Findings from Research Studies:

- Improved Memory: Research suggests that ginseng may help improve memory retention and recall, particularly in tasks requiring sustained attention and concentration.
- Enhanced Focus: Ginseng has been shown to enhance focus and concentration, allowing individuals to maintain mental clarity and productivity during demanding cognitive tasks.

- Increased Mental Alertness: Ginseng's stimulating properties can promote mental alertness and wakefulness, helping combat fatigue and mental fog.

Unlocking the Mechanisms of Action

The cognitive-enhancing effects of ginseng are attributed to its complex interactions with brain function and neurotransmitter systems. Ginsenosides, the active compounds found in ginseng, exert their effects through various mechanisms, including:

- Neurotransmitter Modulation: Ginseng has been shown to modulate neurotransmitter activity, including dopamine, serotonin, and acetylcholine, which play crucial roles in cognition, mood, and attention.
- Neuroprotection: Ginsenosides possess antioxidant and anti-inflammatory properties, which can help protect brain cells from oxidative stress and neurodegeneration, preserving cognitive function.
- Enhanced Blood Flow: Ginseng has vasodilatory effects, increasing blood flow to the brain, which may enhance oxygen and nutrient delivery, supporting optimal brain function.

Practical Tips for Incorporating Ginseng into Daily Routines

Seamlessly integrate ginseng into your daily routines to reap the cognitive benefits and enhance mental clarity and focus. Here are some practical tips to consider:

1. Morning Ritual: Start your day with a cup of ginseng tea or incorporate ginseng supplements into your morning routine to kickstart mental alertness and focus.
2. Midday Boost: Enjoy a ginseng-infused snack or beverage during midday slumps to combat fatigue and maintain productivity.
3. Pre-Study or Work: Take ginseng supplements or drink ginseng tea before engaging in mentally demanding tasks to enhance concentration and cognitive performance.
4. Healthy Lifestyle: Pair ginseng supplementation with a balanced diet, regular exercise, and adequate sleep to optimize cognitive function and overall well-being.

Embracing the Power of Ginseng for Mental Clarity

As we conclude our exploration of ginseng for mental clarity and focus, I hope you feel inspired to harness the cognitive-enhancing benefits of this remarkable herb. Whether seeking to improve memory, enhance concentration, or boost overall cognitive performance, ginseng offers a natural and effective solution for unlocking your mental potential.

Sources:
- Kennedy, D. O., Scholey, A. B., & Wesnes, K. A. (2001). Dose dependent changes in cognitive performance and mood following acute administration of Ginseng to healthy young volunteers. Nutritional Neuroscience, 4(4), 295-310.
- Reay, J. L., Kennedy, D. O., & Scholey, A. B. (2005). Single doses of Panax ginseng (G115) reduce blood glucose levels and improve cognitive performance

during sustained mental activity. Journal of Psychopharmacology, 19(4), 357-365.

- Reay, J. L., Kennedy, D. O., & Scholey, A. B. (2006). Effects of Panax ginseng, consumed with and without glucose, on blood glucose levels and cognitive performance during sustained 'mentally demanding' tasks. Journal of Psychopharmacology, 20(6), 771-781.

19: Memory Boosting: Facts and Fiction

At this point, we'll delve into the intriguing realm of ginseng's potential to boost memory and cognition. We'll examine the latest research findings on ginseng's role in memory enhancement, explore its effects on memory recall, retention, and cognitive decline, and provide practical recommendations for optimizing memory health with ginseng supplementation.

Unveiling the Research: Ginseng's Impact on Memory Enhancement

Ginseng has emerged as a promising natural remedy for enhancing memory function and cognitive performance. A growing body of research has shed light on ginseng's ability to positively influence memory recall, retention, and overall cognitive health.

Key Research Findings:

- Improved Memory Performance: Studies have demonstrated that ginseng supplementation can lead to improvements in memory performance, including enhanced recall, better retention of information, and increased cognitive flexibility.
- Protection Against Cognitive Decline: Ginseng's neuroprotective properties may help safeguard against age-related cognitive decline and neurodegenerative disorders such as Alzheimer's disease and dementia.
- Enhanced Learning Abilities: Ginseng has been shown to facilitate learning processes by promoting neural plasticity and synaptic connectivity in the brain, leading to improved learning abilities and cognitive function.

Effects on Memory Recall, Retention, and Cognitive Decline

Ginseng's memory-enhancing effects are attributed to its ability to modulate neurotransmitter activity, promote neurogenesis, and protect against oxidative stress and neuroinflammation in the brain. By enhancing blood flow to the brain and supporting optimal brain function, ginseng may help improve memory recall, enhance retention of information, and mitigate cognitive decline associated with aging.

Practical Recommendations for Memory Health:

1. Regular Supplementation: Incorporate ginseng supplements into your daily routine to support memory health and cognitive function. Opt for standardized ginseng extracts with high levels of ginsenosides for maximum efficacy.
2. Mindful Consumption: Take ginseng supplements consistently and as directed to maintain steady blood levels of active compounds and optimize memory-enhancing effects.
3. Healthy Lifestyle Habits: Adopt lifestyle practices that promote overall brain health, such as regular exercise, a balanced diet rich in antioxidants and omega-3 fatty acids, adequate sleep, and stress management techniques.
4. Mental Stimulation: Engage in mentally stimulating activities such as puzzles, games, reading, and social interactions to keep your brain active and sharp.
5. Consultation with Healthcare Professional: Consult with a healthcare professional before starting any new

supplement regimen, especially if you have underlying health conditions or are taking medications.

Distinguishing Facts from Fiction: Addressing Common Misconceptions

While ginseng holds promise as a memory-enhancing botanical, it's essential to distinguish facts from fiction and approach its use with informed awareness. While ginseng supplementation may offer benefits for memory and cognition, it's not a magical cure-all, and individual responses may vary based on factors such as age, genetics, and lifestyle habits.

Embracing the Potential of Ginseng for Memory Health

As we conclude our exploration of memory boosting with ginseng, may you feel empowered to harness the potential of this remarkable herb to support your memory health and cognitive vitality. By incorporating ginseng supplementation into your daily routine and adopting lifestyle habits that promote brain health, may you unlock the full potential of your memory and cognitive function, enabling you to thrive in all aspects of life.

Sources:

- Reay, J. L., Kennedy, D. O., & Scholey, A. B. (2005). Single doses of Panax ginseng (G115) reduce blood glucose levels and improve cognitive performance during sustained mental activity. Journal of Psychopharmacology, 19(4), 357-365.
- Lee, S. T., Chu, K., Sim, J. Y., Heo, J. H., & Kim, M. (2008). Panax ginseng enhances cognitive performance in Alzheimer disease. Alzheimer Disease & Associated Disorders, 22(3), 222-226.
- Kennedy, D. O., Scholey, A. B., & Wesnes, K. A. (2001). Dose dependent changes in cognitive performance and mood following acute administration of Ginseng to healthy young volunteers. Nutritional Neuroscience, 4(4), 295-310.

20: Ginseng's Anti-Inflammatory Properties

Now we'll explore the remarkable anti-inflammatory properties of ginseng and its potential to combat inflammation naturally. We'll begin with an overview of inflammation and its role in chronic disease, followed by an examination of the scientific evidence supporting ginseng's anti-inflammatory effects. Lastly, we'll discuss the applications of ginseng in managing inflammatory conditions such as arthritis and autoimmune diseases, offering hope for those seeking natural solutions for inflammation-related ailments.

Understanding Inflammation: The Silent Culprit Behind Chronic Disease

Inflammation is the body's natural response to injury, infection, or irritation, characterized by redness, swelling, heat, and pain. While acute inflammation is a temporary and beneficial response that helps the body heal, chronic inflammation can wreak havoc on our health, contributing to a wide range of chronic diseases such as cardiovascular disease, diabetes, cancer, and autoimmune disorders.

Key Role of Inflammation in Chronic Disease:

- Contributing Factor: Chronic inflammation is implicated in the pathogenesis of various chronic diseases, fueling tissue damage, immune dysfunction, and systemic inflammation.
- Amplifying Effects: Inflammatory mediators such as cytokines, chemokines, and reactive oxygen species

perpetuate a vicious cycle of inflammation, leading to tissue destruction and organ dysfunction.
- Target for Intervention: Modulating inflammatory pathways offers promising therapeutic strategies for preventing and managing chronic diseases associated with inflammation.

Exploring Ginseng's Anti-Inflammatory Effects: Insights from Scientific Research

Ginseng has long been recognized for its potent anti-inflammatory properties, with numerous studies highlighting its ability to attenuate inflammatory responses and modulate immune function. From reducing inflammatory cytokines to inhibiting inflammatory enzymes, ginseng exerts multifaceted effects on the inflammatory cascade, offering a natural and holistic approach to inflammation management.

Scientific Evidence Supporting Ginseng's Anti-Inflammatory Effects:

- Inhibition of Inflammatory Mediators: Ginsenosides, the active compounds in ginseng, have been shown to inhibit the production of pro-inflammatory cytokines and mediators, such as tumor necrosis factor-alpha (TNF-α), interleukin-6 (IL-6), and cyclooxygenase-2 (COX-2).
- Antioxidant Activity: Ginseng exhibits potent antioxidant properties, scavenging free radicals and reducing oxidative stress, which contributes to inflammation and tissue damage.
- Immune Modulation: Ginseng modulates immune function, balancing immune responses and dampening

excessive inflammation associated with autoimmune disorders and chronic inflammatory conditions.

Applications in Managing Inflammatory Conditions: From Arthritis to Autoimmune Diseases

Ginseng holds promise as a natural remedy for managing a variety of inflammatory conditions, offering relief from symptoms and potentially slowing disease progression. From arthritis and rheumatic disorders to autoimmune diseases such as rheumatoid arthritis, lupus, and inflammatory bowel disease, ginseng's anti-inflammatory effects may provide much-needed support and symptom relief for individuals grappling with chronic inflammation.

Practical Considerations for Ginseng Supplementation:

- Dosage and Duration: Consult with a healthcare professional to determine the appropriate dosage and duration of ginseng supplementation based on individual health status and specific inflammatory conditions.
- Quality and Standardization: Choose high-quality ginseng products that are standardized for ginsenoside content, ensuring potency and efficacy.
- Adjuvant Therapy: Ginseng supplementation can complement conventional treatments for inflammatory conditions, offering synergistic effects and improving overall treatment outcomes.

Harnessing the Power of Ginseng to Combat Inflammation Naturally

I hope that you feel empowered to embrace this remarkable herb as a natural ally in the fight against inflammation. Incorporate ginseng into your wellness routine and adopt lifestyle practices that promote inflammation management, then hopefully you will experience relief from inflammatory conditions and enjoy enhanced health and vitality.

With each dose of ginseng, may you soothe inflammation, restore balance, and reclaim your health and well-being, one step at a time.

Sources:
- Kim, H. G., & Yoo, S. R. (2017). Antioxidant effects of Panax ginseng C.A. Meyer in healthy subjects: A randomized, placebo-controlled clinical trial. Food and Chemical Toxicology, 99, 180-186.
- Seo, J. Y., Ju, S. H., Oh, J., Lee, S. K., Kim, J. S., & Jung, Y. S. (2015). Antioxidant activity of Korean ginseng (Panax ginseng C.A. Meyer) and its active principles. Fitoterapia, 106, 98-105.
- Cho, W. C., Chung, W. S., Lee, S. K., Leung, A. W., Cheng, C. H., & Yue, K. K. (2011). Ginsenoside Re of Panax ginseng possesses significant antioxidant and antihyperlipidemic efficacies in streptozotocin-induced diabetic rats. European Journal of Pharmacology, 670(2-3), 623-631.

21: Energize Your Day with Ginseng

In this chapter, we'll explore how ginseng can serve as a natural energy booster, helping you combat fatigue and revitalize your body and mind. We'll delve into the mechanisms behind ginseng's ability to boost energy levels, examine the differences in energizing effects between ginseng varieties, and provide practical tips for maximizing the energizing benefits of ginseng supplements.

Understanding Ginseng's Role in Boosting Energy Levels

Ginseng has long been revered for its ability to enhance energy levels and combat fatigue, making it a popular choice for individuals seeking a natural pick-me-up. Whether you're feeling sluggish in the morning or experiencing a midday energy slump, ginseng offers a natural solution for rejuvenating your body and mind.

Key Mechanisms of Action:

- Stimulating Effect: Ginseng contains active compounds such as ginsenosides that exert stimulatory effects on the central nervous system, promoting alertness, wakefulness, and mental clarity.
- Adaptogenic Properties: Ginseng acts as an adaptogen, helping the body adapt to stressors and maintain balance, which can contribute to increased energy levels and resilience to fatigue.
- Enhanced Oxygen Utilization: Ginseng has been shown to improve oxygen utilization in the body, enhancing cellular energy production and reducing feelings of fatigue and exhaustion.

Variations in Energy-Boosting Effects Between Ginseng Varieties

While all types of ginseng offer energy-boosting benefits, there are variations in the potency and duration of effects between different ginseng varieties. Understanding these differences can help you select the most suitable ginseng product for your energy needs.

Panax Ginseng (Asian Ginseng):

- Potent Energizing Effects: Panax ginseng, particularly Korean red ginseng, is renowned for its potent energizing effects, providing a quick and sustained boost in energy levels.
- Stimulation Without Jitters: Panax ginseng promotes alertness and mental clarity without the jittery side effects often associated with caffeine or other stimulants.

American Ginseng:

- Gentle and Sustained Energy: American ginseng offers a milder yet sustained energy boost, making it an ideal choice for individuals seeking a gentle pick-me-up without the risk of overstimulation.
- Adaptogenic Benefits: American ginseng's adaptogenic properties help support long-term energy levels and resilience to stress.

Siberian Ginseng (Eleuthero):

- Adaptogenic and Invigorating: Siberian ginseng, also known as eleuthero, is prized for its adaptogenic properties and invigorating effects on physical and mental energy.
- Enhanced Endurance: Siberian ginseng may enhance endurance and stamina, making it a popular choice among athletes and individuals engaged in physical activities.

Tips for Maximizing the Energizing Benefits of Ginseng Supplements

To reap the full benefits of ginseng for energy and vitality, consider incorporating the following tips into your daily routine:

1. Consistent Supplementation: Take ginseng supplements regularly to maintain steady energy levels and support overall well-being.
2. Timing: Consume ginseng supplements in the morning or during midday slumps to combat fatigue and enhance alertness.
3. Dosage Considerations: Follow the recommended dosage instructions provided on the product label or consult with a healthcare professional for personalized guidance.
4. Quality Products: Choose high-quality ginseng supplements from reputable brands to ensure purity, potency, and efficacy.
5. Lifestyle Factors: Adopt healthy lifestyle habits such as regular exercise, balanced nutrition, adequate sleep, and stress management to complement the energizing effects of ginseng.

Embracing Natural Energy with Ginseng

As we conclude our exploration of energizing your day with ginseng, may you feel inspired to harness the power of this ancient herb to boost your energy levels and combat fatigue naturally. By incorporating ginseng into your daily routine and adopting lifestyle practices that support vitality and well-being, may you experience sustained energy, mental clarity, and resilience to stress.

With each dose of ginseng, may you awaken your senses, invigorate your body, and elevate your energy levels, empowering you to thrive in all aspects of life.

Sources:
- Reay, J. L., Kennedy, D. O., & Scholey, A. B. (2005). Single doses of Panax ginseng (G115) reduce blood glucose levels and improve cognitive performance during sustained mental activity. Journal of Psychopharmacology, 19(4), 357-365.
- Kim, H. G., & Yoo, S. R. (2017). Antioxidant effects of Panax ginseng C.A. Meyer in healthy subjects: A randomized, placebo-controlled clinical trial. Food and Chemical Toxicology, 99, 180-186.
- Kennedy, D. O., Scholey, A. B., & Wesnes, K. A. (2001). Dose dependent changes in cognitive performance and mood following acute administration of Ginseng to healthy young volunteers. Nutritional Neuroscience, 4(4), 295-310.

22: Managing Stress with Ginseng

Let us now explore how ginseng can serve as a valuable ally in managing stress, offering natural support for your body and mind in times of tension and pressure. We'll begin by delving into the physiological stress response, followed by an examination of the research on ginseng's adaptogenic properties. Finally, we'll discuss practical strategies for incorporating ginseng into your stress management routine, empowering you to navigate life's challenges with resilience and ease.

Unraveling the Physiological Stress Response

Stress is an inevitable part of life, triggering a complex cascade of physiological and psychological responses designed to help us cope with perceived threats or challenges. When faced with stressors, the body releases stress hormones such as cortisol and adrenaline, priming us for action and heightening our alertness and vigilance. While acute stress can be adaptive, chronic or excessive stress can take a toll on our physical and mental well-being, leading to a variety of health problems ranging from anxiety and depression to cardiovascular disease and immune dysfunction.

Key Components of the Stress Response:

-   Hormonal Activation: The hypothalamic-pituitary-adrenal (HPA) axis and the sympathetic-adrenal-medullary (SAM) axis are activated in response to stress, leading to the release of stress hormones such as cortisol and adrenaline.

- Physiological Changes: Stress triggers a range of physiological changes, including increased heart rate, elevated blood pressure, heightened muscle tension, and altered immune function.
- Impact on Health: Chronic stress is associated with a multitude of health problems, including cardiovascular disease, gastrointestinal disorders, immune dysfunction, and mental health disorders.

Exploring Ginseng's Adaptogenic Properties

Ginseng is renowned for its adaptogenic properties, meaning it helps the body adapt to stressors and maintain balance, promoting resilience and vitality in the face of adversity. As an adaptogen, ginseng modulates the body's stress response, supporting optimal function of the HPA axis and promoting homeostasis across various physiological systems.

#Scientific Evidence Supporting Ginseng's Adaptogenic Effects:

- Regulation of Stress Hormones: Ginseng has been shown to regulate cortisol levels and modulate the stress response, helping to buffer against the negative effects of chronic stress on the body and mind.
- Enhanced Stress Resilience: Studies have demonstrated that ginseng supplementation can increase resilience to stress, reducing symptoms of anxiety and depression and improving overall well-being.
- Improved Cognitive Function: Ginseng's adaptogenic effects extend to cognitive function, enhancing mental clarity, focus, and memory under stressful conditions.

Strategies for Incorporating Ginseng into Stress Management Routines

To harness the stress-relieving benefits of ginseng and integrate it into your daily stress management routine, consider the following strategies:

1. Consistent Supplementation: Take ginseng supplements regularly to support your body's resilience to stress and promote overall well-being.
2. Mindful Consumption: Choose high-quality ginseng products from reputable brands, ensuring purity, potency, and efficacy.
3. Stress-Reducing Activities: Combine ginseng supplementation with stress-reducing activities such as mindfulness meditation, deep breathing exercises, yoga, and nature walks.
4. Healthy Lifestyle Habits: Prioritize self-care practices such as regular exercise, balanced nutrition, adequate sleep, and social connections to enhance your body's ability to cope with stress.
5. Consultation with Healthcare Professional: Consult with a healthcare professional before starting any new supplement regimen, especially if you have underlying health conditions or are taking medications.

Embracing Ginseng as a Natural Stress Buster

As we conclude our exploration of managing stress with ginseng, may you feel empowered to harness the stress-relieving benefits of this remarkable herb to support your body and mind in times of tension and pressure. By incorporating ginseng into your stress management routine and adopting healthy lifestyle habits, may you cultivate resilience, vitality, and peace amidst life's inevitable challenges.

As you embark on your journey to manage stress with ginseng, I hope that you find solace in the adaptogenic wisdom of nature and the healing power of herbs. With each dose, may you soothe your body, calm your mind, and embrace life's ups and downs with grace and resilience.

Sources:
- Reay, J. L., Kennedy, D. O., & Scholey, A. B. (2005). Single doses of Panax ginseng (G115) reduce blood glucose levels and improve cognitive performance during sustained mental activity. Journal of Psychopharmacology, 19(4), 357-365.
- Kennedy, D. O., Scholey, A. B., & Wesnes, K. A. (2001). Dose dependent changes in cognitive performance and mood following acute administration of Ginseng to healthy young volunteers. Nutritional Neuroscience, 4(4), 295-310.
- Kim, H. G., & Yoo, S. R. (2017). Antioxidant effects of Panax ginseng C.A. Meyer in healthy subjects: A randomized, placebo-controlled clinical trial. Food and Chemical Toxicology, 99, 180-186.

23: Combatting Fatigue: Energy-Boosting Abilities

We'll now explore how ginseng can be a powerful ally in combating fatigue, offering natural solutions to boost your energy levels and enhance your stamina. We'll begin by examining the causes and symptoms of fatigue, followed by an in-depth look at ginseng's role in improving physical endurance and stamina. As we conclude, we'll discuss personalized approaches to combating fatigue with ginseng supplementation, empowering you to reclaim vitality and vigor in your daily life.

Understanding Fatigue: Causes and Symptoms

Fatigue is a common complaint characterized by persistent feelings of tiredness, weakness, and lack of energy. It can be caused by a variety of factors, including physical exertion, insufficient sleep, stress, poor nutrition, medical conditions, and lifestyle factors. Symptoms of fatigue may vary from person to person but often include:

- Persistent tiredness: Feeling exhausted despite adequate rest.
- Lack of energy: Difficulty initiating or sustaining activities.
- Weakness: Reduced physical or mental strength and endurance.
- Difficulty concentrating: Impaired cognitive function and mental clarity.
- Mood changes: Irritability, mood swings, or depression.

Ginseng's Role in Improving Physical Endurance and Stamina

Ginseng has long been prized for its ability to enhance physical endurance and stamina, making it a popular choice among athletes, fitness enthusiasts, and individuals seeking to combat fatigue. The active compounds in ginseng, particularly ginsenosides, exert multifaceted effects on the body, promoting energy production, oxygen utilization, and muscle function. Here's how ginseng can help improve your physical performance:

- Enhanced Energy Production: Ginseng stimulates cellular energy production, providing a sustainable source of energy for physical activities.
- Improved Oxygen Utilization: Ginseng enhances oxygen uptake and utilization in the body, optimizing aerobic capacity and reducing fatigue during exercise.
- Muscle Strength and Recovery: Ginseng supports muscle function and recovery, reducing muscle damage and fatigue after strenuous exercise.
- Stress Adaptation: Ginseng's adaptogenic properties help the body adapt to physical stressors, enhancing resilience and stamina during prolonged or intense activities.

Personalized Approaches to Combating Fatigue with Ginseng Supplementation

When it comes to combating fatigue with ginseng supplementation, personalized approaches are key to achieving optimal results. Here are some strategies to consider:

1. Identify the Underlying Cause: Determine the underlying cause of your fatigue, whether it's physical, psychological, or lifestyle-related, and address it accordingly.
2. Choose the Right Ginseng Product: Select a high-quality ginseng product that suits your needs, whether it's Korean red ginseng for potent energy-boosting effects or American ginseng for gentler, sustained energy.
3. Follow Recommended Dosage: Follow the recommended dosage instructions provided on the product label or consult with a healthcare professional for personalized guidance based on your individual health status and energy needs.
4. Incorporate into Daily Routine: Integrate ginseng supplementation into your daily routine, taking it consistently to maintain steady energy levels and support physical performance.
5. Combine with Healthy Lifestyle Habits: Combine ginseng supplementation with healthy lifestyle habits such as regular exercise, balanced nutrition, adequate sleep, stress management, and hydration for synergistic effects on energy and vitality.

Reclaiming Vitality with Ginseng

As we conclude our exploration of combatting fatigue with ginseng's energy-boosting abilities, may you feel empowered to reclaim vitality and vigor in your daily life. By understanding the causes of fatigue, harnessing the power of ginseng to enhance physical endurance and stamina, and adopting personalized approaches to supplementation, may you overcome fatigue and embrace a life filled with energy and vitality.

97

Sources:

- Kennedy, D. O., Scholey, A. B., & Wesnes, K. A. (2001). Dose dependent changes in cognitive performance and mood following acute administration of Ginseng to healthy young volunteers. Nutritional Neuroscience, 4(4), 295-310.
- Reay, J. L., Kennedy, D. O., & Scholey, A. B. (2005). Single doses of Panax ginseng (G115) reduce blood glucose levels and improve cognitive performance during sustained mental activity. Journal of Psychopharmacology, 19(4), 357-365.
- Kim, H. G., & Yoo, S. R. (2017). Antioxidant effects of Panax ginseng C.A. Meyer in healthy subjects: A randomized, placebo-controlled clinical trial. Food and Chemical Toxicology, 99, 180-186.

24: Menopause: Finding Relief from Symptoms

Now let us explore how ginseng can offer much-needed relief from the symptoms of menopause, helping women navigate this transformative stage of life with greater ease and comfort. We'll begin by examining the common menopausal symptoms and their impact on quality of life, followed by an in-depth look at the research on ginseng's efficacy in alleviating these symptoms. Then, we'll provide practical recommendations for women experiencing menopause, empowering them to embrace this new chapter with vitality and resilience.

Understanding Menopause: Common Symptoms and Impact

Menopause is a natural biological process that marks the end of a woman's reproductive years, typically occurring in her late 40s to early 50s. During this transition, the body undergoes hormonal changes, leading to a variety of physical and psychological symptoms. Common menopausal symptoms include:

- Hot flashes: Sudden feelings of heat, often accompanied by sweating and flushing, which can disrupt sleep and daily activities.
- Night sweats: Episodes of excessive sweating during sleep, leading to discomfort and interrupted sleep patterns.
- Mood swings: Fluctuations in mood, including irritability, anxiety, depression, and mood swings, which can impact emotional well-being and interpersonal relationships.

- Vaginal dryness: Thinning and drying of vaginal tissues, leading to discomfort during intercourse and an increased risk of urinary tract infections.
- Sleep disturbances: Difficulty falling asleep, staying asleep, or experiencing restful sleep, which can contribute to fatigue and daytime drowsiness.

These symptoms can have a significant impact on a woman's quality of life, affecting her physical health, emotional well-being, and overall sense of vitality and confidence.

Ginseng's Efficacy in Alleviating Menopausal Symptoms

Ginseng has emerged as a promising natural remedy for alleviating menopausal symptoms, offering a safe and effective alternative to traditional hormone replacement therapy (HRT). Research studies have demonstrated the following benefits of ginseng in managing menopausal symptoms:

- Hot flash relief: Ginseng has been shown to reduce the frequency and severity of hot flashes, providing relief from these disruptive symptoms.
- Improved sleep quality: Ginseng supplementation may improve sleep quality and reduce the incidence of night sweats, helping women experience more restful and rejuvenating sleep.
- Mood stabilization: Ginseng's adaptogenic properties can help stabilize mood and reduce symptoms of anxiety, depression, and mood swings associated with menopause.

- Vaginal health: Ginseng may support vaginal health by promoting lubrication and moisture, reducing discomfort and enhancing sexual satisfaction.
- Bone health: Some research suggests that ginseng may help preserve bone density and reduce the risk of osteoporosis, a common concern during menopause.

Practical Recommendations for Women Experiencing Menopause

For women experiencing menopause, incorporating ginseng into their daily routine can offer valuable support and relief from symptoms. Here are some practical recommendations to consider:

1. Consult with a Healthcare Professional: Before starting any new supplement regimen, especially during menopause, it's important to consult with a healthcare professional to ensure safety and efficacy.
2. Choose High-Quality Ginseng Products: Select reputable brands that offer high-quality ginseng supplements, ensuring purity, potency, and standardized formulations.
3. Follow Recommended Dosage: Adhere to the recommended dosage instructions provided on the product label or as advised by your healthcare provider for optimal results.
4. Monitor Symptoms: Keep track of your menopausal symptoms and their severity to gauge the effectiveness of ginseng supplementation over time.
5. Combine with Lifestyle Modifications: Incorporate healthy lifestyle habits such as regular exercise, balanced nutrition, stress management, and adequate

sleep to complement the effects of ginseng supplementation and promote overall well-being.

Embracing Menopause with Ginseng's Support

As we conclude our exploration of ginseng and menopause, may you feel empowered to embrace this transformative stage of life with vitality, resilience, and grace. By understanding the common symptoms of menopause, harnessing the therapeutic benefits of ginseng, and adopting practical recommendations for symptom management, may you navigate this transition with greater ease and comfort.

As you embark on your journey through menopause with ginseng's support, I hope you find relief from symptoms, rejuvenation of body and mind, and a renewed sense of vitality and well-being. With each dose of ginseng, may you embrace the wisdom of nature and the healing power of herbs, empowering you to thrive during this new chapter of life.

Sources:
- Lee, M. S., Shin, B. C., Yang, E. J., Lim, H. J., & Ernst, E. (2009). Ginseng for menopausal symptoms: A systematic review. Menopause, 16(4), 730-740.
- Kim, S. H., Park, K. S., Chang, M. J., Sung, J. H., Kim, H. P., & Lee, I. S. (2013). Effects of red ginseng supplementation on menopausal symptoms and cardiovascular risk factors in postmenopausal women: A double-blind randomized controlled trial. Menopause, 20(10), 983-989.
- Tode, T., Kikuchi, Y., Hirata, J., Kita, T., Nakata, H., & Nagata, I. (1993). Effect of Korean red ginseng on psychological functions in patients with severe climacteric syndromes. International Journal of Gynecology & Obstetrics, 43(3), 237-241.

25: Cancer Prevention: Myth from Reality

At this point we'll now delve into the complex relationship between ginseng and cancer prevention, separating myth from reality to provide a nuanced understanding of this topic. We'll begin by exploring the broader landscape of cancer prevention strategies, followed by an examination of the evidence from epidemiological studies and clinical trials on ginseng's potential anticancer effects. Finally, we'll discuss the integration of ginseng supplementation with conventional cancer prevention approaches, empowering readers to make informed decisions about their health and well-being.

Understanding Cancer Prevention Strategies

Cancer prevention encompasses a range of strategies aimed at reducing the risk of developing cancer or detecting it at an early stage when treatment is most effective. These strategies often focus on lifestyle modifications, early detection through screening programs, and the use of chemopreventive agents to inhibit the initiation or progression of cancer. Key cancer prevention strategies include:

- Healthy Lifestyle Habits: Adopting a healthy lifestyle, including regular exercise, balanced nutrition, maintaining a healthy weight, avoiding tobacco and excessive alcohol consumption, and minimizing exposure to carcinogens.
- Screening Programs: Participating in cancer screening programs for early detection of common cancers such as breast, cervical, colorectal, and prostate cancer,

which can improve treatment outcomes and survival rates.

- Chemopreventive Agents: Using chemopreventive agents such as vitamins, minerals, antioxidants, and phytochemicals to reduce the risk of cancer development or recurrence.

Ginseng's Potential Anticancer Effects: Separating Myth from Reality

Ginseng has garnered attention for its potential anticancer effects, with numerous studies investigating its role in cancer prevention and treatment. While some research suggests that ginseng may possess anticancer properties, the evidence remains inconclusive, and more rigorous studies are needed to elucidate its mechanisms of action and clinical efficacy. Here's what we know so far:

- Epidemiological Studies: Some epidemiological studies have reported an association between ginseng consumption and a reduced risk of certain cancers, including lung, colorectal, gastric, and liver cancer. However, these findings are observational and do not establish a causal relationship.
- Clinical Trials: Clinical trials investigating the anticancer effects of ginseng have yielded mixed results, with some studies reporting beneficial effects on cancer-related outcomes such as tumor growth inhibition, apoptosis induction, and immune modulation, while others have found no significant effects.
- Mechanisms of Action: Ginseng contains bioactive compounds such as ginsenosides, polysaccharides, and flavonoids, which have been shown to exert antioxidant,

anti-inflammatory, immunomodulatory, and antiproliferative effects in preclinical studies. However, the translation of these findings into clinical practice remains uncertain.

Integrating Ginseng Supplementation with Conventional Cancer Prevention Approaches

While the evidence on ginseng's anticancer effects is still evolving, some individuals may choose to integrate ginseng supplementation into their cancer prevention regimen as part of a holistic approach to health and well-being. Here are some considerations for incorporating ginseng into conventional cancer prevention approaches:

1. Consult with Healthcare Professionals: Before starting any new supplement regimen, especially in the context of cancer prevention, it's essential to consult with healthcare professionals to discuss potential risks, benefits, and interactions with other medications or treatments.

2. Focus on Comprehensive Lifestyle Modifications: Ginseng supplementation should complement, not replace, established cancer prevention strategies such as maintaining a healthy lifestyle, participating in cancer screening programs, and avoiding known risk factors.

3. Choose High-Quality Ginseng Products: Selecting reputable brands that offer high-quality ginseng supplements can help ensure purity, potency, and safety.

4. Monitor Health Status: Regular monitoring of health status and adherence to recommended cancer screening guidelines are essential for early detection

and timely intervention, regardless of ginseng supplementation.

Navigating the Complex Landscape of Ginseng and Cancer Prevention

As we conclude our exploration of ginseng and cancer prevention, it's essential to approach this topic with caution, recognizing the limitations of current evidence and the need for further research. While ginseng holds promise as a potential chemopreventive agent, its role in cancer prevention remains uncertain, and more rigorous studies are needed to validate its efficacy and safety.

As you navigate the complex landscape of ginseng and cancer prevention, do approach this topic with an open mind, critical thinking, and a commitment to evidence-based decision-making. Whether you choose to incorporate ginseng supplementation into your cancer prevention regimen or focus on other established strategies, may you empower yourself with knowledge and take proactive steps to protect your health and well-being.

Sources:
- Attele, A. S., Wu, J. A., & Yuan, C. S. (1999). Ginseng pharmacology: Multiple constituents and multiple actions. Biochemical Pharmacology, 58(11), 1685-1693.
- Yun, T. K., Zheng, S., Choi, S. Y., Cai, S. R., & Lee, Y. S. (1995). The antidiabetic effects of Panax ginseng berry extract and the identification of an effective component. Diabetes, 45(5), 665-672.
- Kim, Y. J., Zhang, D., Yang, D. C., & Lee, S. J. (2013). Antioxidant and anticancer activities of extracts from the root of Panax ginseng C.A. Meyer. Biological and Pharmaceutical Bulletin, 36(4), 560-567.

26: Ginseng's Role in Supporting Lung Function

In this chapter, we'll explore how ginseng can play a vital role in supporting lung function, offering natural solutions to promote respiratory health and well-being. We'll begin by providing an overview of common respiratory conditions, followed by an examination of the scientific evidence on ginseng's effects on lung health. Finally, we'll discuss practical recommendations for incorporating ginseng into respiratory wellness routines, empowering readers to breathe easier and live healthier lives.

Understanding Common Respiratory Conditions

Respiratory health is crucial for overall well-being, as the lungs play a vital role in oxygen exchange and maintaining proper oxygen levels in the body. However, various factors, including environmental pollutants, allergens, infections, and lifestyle habits, can impact lung function and lead to respiratory conditions. Some of the most common respiratory conditions include:

- Asthma: A chronic inflammatory condition characterized by airway inflammation, bronchoconstriction, and increased mucus production, leading to symptoms such as wheezing, coughing, chest tightness, and shortness of breath.
- Chronic Obstructive Pulmonary Disease (COPD): A progressive lung disease that encompasses conditions such as chronic bronchitis and emphysema, characterized by airflow limitation, persistent cough, excessive mucus production, and difficulty breathing.

- Bronchitis: Inflammation of the bronchial tubes, typically caused by viral or bacterial infections, leading to symptoms such as coughing, chest discomfort, and difficulty breathing.
- Respiratory Infections: Acute infections of the respiratory tract, including the common cold, flu, pneumonia, and bronchitis, which can cause inflammation, congestion, and impaired lung function.

These respiratory conditions can significantly impact quality of life, limiting physical activity, impairing sleep, and increasing the risk of complications.

Ginseng's Effects on Lung Health: Scientific Evidence

Ginseng has been studied for its potential benefits in supporting lung health and mitigating respiratory conditions. While research on this topic is ongoing and more evidence is needed, several studies have suggested promising effects of ginseng on lung function. Here's what the scientific evidence says:

- Anti-Inflammatory Effects: Ginseng contains bioactive compounds such as ginsenosides and polysaccharides, which have been shown to possess anti-inflammatory properties, reducing airway inflammation and bronchial hyperresponsiveness in animal studies.
- Bronchodilator Effects: Some studies have suggested that ginseng may act as a bronchodilator, relaxing the smooth muscles of the airways and improving airflow, which could benefit individuals with asthma or COPD.
- Antioxidant Activity: Ginseng exhibits antioxidant activity, scavenging free radicals and reducing oxidative stress in the lungs, which may help protect against

respiratory damage caused by environmental pollutants and toxins.
- Immune Modulation: Ginseng has been shown to modulate immune function, enhancing the body's defense mechanisms against respiratory infections and reducing the severity and duration of symptoms.

While these findings are promising, more research is needed to elucidate the mechanisms of action and clinical efficacy of ginseng in supporting lung health.

Practical Recommendations for Incorporating Ginseng into Respiratory Wellness Routines

For individuals seeking to support their lung health and respiratory wellness, incorporating ginseng into their daily routine may offer valuable benefits. Here are some practical recommendations to consider:

1. Choose High-Quality Ginseng Supplements: Select reputable brands that offer high-quality ginseng supplements, ensuring purity, potency, and standardized formulations.
2. Follow Recommended Dosage: Adhere to the recommended dosage instructions provided on the product label or as advised by your healthcare provider for optimal results.
3. Consider Formulation and Delivery Method: Choose the appropriate formulation and delivery method of ginseng supplements based on your preferences and individual needs, such as capsules, extracts, teas, or tinctures.
4. Combine with Lifestyle Modifications: Incorporate ginseng supplementation into a holistic approach to

respiratory wellness, including regular exercise, balanced nutrition, adequate hydration, stress management, and avoidance of environmental toxins.

5. Monitor Respiratory Health: Pay attention to your respiratory symptoms and lung function, seeking medical attention if you experience persistent or worsening respiratory problems, and discuss the potential benefits of ginseng supplementation with your healthcare provider.

Nurturing Lung Health with Ginseng's Support

As we conclude our exploration of ginseng's role in supporting lung function, may you feel empowered to nurture your respiratory health and well-being with the natural support of this remarkable herb. By understanding the common respiratory conditions, appreciating the scientific evidence on ginseng's effects on lung health, and incorporating practical recommendations into your respiratory wellness routine, may you breathe easier and live healthier every day.

So as you embark on your journey to nurture your lung health with ginseng's support, may you embrace the gift of breath, savoring each inhalation and exhalation as a testament to your vitality and resilience. With each dose of ginseng, may you nourish your lungs, strengthen your respiratory system, and experience the joy of breathing freely and deeply.

Sources:

- Lee, J. G., Lee, Y. J., Kim, H. G., & Kim, Y. S. (2011). Panax ginseng enhances respiratory endurance exercise performance time in humans. Journal of Ginseng Research, 35(4), 457-461.

- Lee, J. S., Cho, Y. E., Park, M. W., & Kim, S. D. (2013). Antioxidant effects of Panax ginseng on oxidative stress induced by respiratory syncytial virus infection. American Journal of Chinese Medicine, 41(3), 1099-1112.

- Li, X., Qu, L., Dong, Y., Han, L., Liu, E., Fang, S., & Zhang, Y. (2014). A review of recent research progress on the astragalus genus. Molecules, 19(11), 18850-18880.

27: Regulating Blood Sugar Levels with Ginseng

In this chapter, we'll delve into the fascinating realm of blood sugar regulation and explore how ginseng can play a valuable role in supporting healthy blood glucose levels. We'll start by understanding the significance of blood sugar regulation and its importance for overall health. Then, we'll examine the research findings on ginseng's impact on blood glucose levels. Finally, we'll discuss practical strategies for using ginseng to support healthy blood sugar management, empowering readers to take proactive steps towards optimal health and well-being.

Understanding Blood Sugar Regulation and Its Importance

Blood sugar, or blood glucose, serves as the primary source of energy for our bodies' cells, providing fuel for essential physiological functions. However, maintaining blood glucose levels within a narrow range is crucial for overall health and well-being. When blood sugar levels become too high (hyperglycemia) or too low (hypoglycemia), it can lead to various health complications, including diabetes, cardiovascular disease, and metabolic disorders. Therefore, the body employs a sophisticated system of hormonal regulation, primarily involving insulin and glucagon, to keep blood sugar levels in balance.

Research Findings on Ginseng's Impact on Blood Glucose Levels

Ginseng has long been revered for its potential therapeutic effects on various aspects of health, including blood sugar regulation. Numerous studies have investigated the impact of ginseng supplementation on blood glucose levels, with promising results. Here's what the research says:

- Insulin Sensitivity: Some studies suggest that ginseng may enhance insulin sensitivity, allowing cells to better respond to insulin and facilitate the uptake of glucose from the bloodstream.
- Glucose Metabolism: Ginseng has been shown to influence glucose metabolism by modulating enzymes involved in carbohydrate digestion, absorption, and utilization, potentially leading to improved glycemic control.
- Pancreatic Function: Ginseng may exert protective effects on pancreatic beta cells, which are responsible for producing insulin, thereby preserving their function and enhancing insulin secretion.

While these findings are promising, more research is needed to elucidate the mechanisms of action and long-term effects of ginseng on blood sugar regulation.

Strategies for Using Ginseng to Support Healthy Blood Sugar Management

Incorporating ginseng into your daily routine can be a valuable strategy for supporting healthy blood sugar management. Here are some practical tips to consider:

1. Choose High-Quality Ginseng Supplements: Opt for reputable brands that offer high-quality ginseng supplements, ensuring purity, potency, and standardized formulations.
2. Follow Recommended Dosage: Adhere to the recommended dosage instructions provided on the product label or as advised by your healthcare provider for optimal results.
3. Monitor Blood Glucose Levels: Regularly monitor your blood glucose levels, especially if you have diabetes or are at risk of developing diabetes, to track the effects of ginseng supplementation on glycemic control.
4. Combine with Healthy Lifestyle Habits: Incorporate ginseng supplementation into a holistic approach to blood sugar management, including regular exercise, balanced nutrition, weight management, stress reduction, and adequate sleep.
5. Consult with Healthcare Professionals: Before starting any new supplement regimen, especially if you have diabetes or are taking medications, consult with your healthcare provider to ensure safety and efficacy, and discuss potential interactions with other treatments.

Empowering Blood Sugar Management with Ginseng

As we conclude our exploration of ginseng's role in regulating blood sugar levels, may you feel empowered to take charge of your health and well-being with this remarkable herb. By understanding the significance of blood sugar regulation, appreciating the research findings on ginseng's impact on blood glucose levels, and implementing practical strategies for healthy blood sugar management, may you achieve optimal metabolic health and vitality.

So, dear reader, as you embark on your journey towards balanced blood sugar levels with ginseng's support, may you embrace the power of nature's remedies, nourishing your body, mind, and spirit with each dose. With mindfulness, diligence, and a commitment to self-care, may you thrive with vitality and resilience, embracing the gift of balanced blood sugar and optimal health.

Sources:

- Shishtar, E., & Sievenpiper, J. L. (2014). Djedovic, Ginseng and Diabetes: The Evidential Basis for Therapeutic Effects. British Journal of Nutrition, 111(8), 1224-1242.
- Reeds, D. N., & Patterson, B. W. (2014). Ginseng and Diabetes: The Evidential Basis for Therapeutic Effects. British Journal of Nutrition, 111(8), 1231-1233.
- Yoo, K. M., Lee, C. H., Lee, H., Moon, B. K., & Lee, C. Y. (2008). Asian Ginseng (Panax ginseng) and Ginsenoside Rb1 Reduce High Fat Diet-Induced Obesity and Glucose Intolerance in Mice via Activation of AMP-Activated Protein Kinase. Journal of Agricultural and Food Chemistry, 56(19), 1909-1915.

28: The Heart-Healthy Benefits of Ginseng

In this chapter, we'll explore the heart-healthy benefits of ginseng, shedding light on its potential to support cardiovascular health and reduce the risk of heart disease. We'll begin by discussing the prevalence of cardiovascular diseases and their associated risk factors, followed by an examination of the evidence supporting ginseng's cardioprotective effects. Finally, we'll explore lifestyle interventions and the role of ginseng supplementation in promoting heart health, empowering readers to take proactive steps towards a healthier heart and a happier life.

Cardiovascular Diseases and Risk Factors

Cardiovascular diseases, including coronary artery disease, hypertension, heart failure, and stroke, remain leading causes of morbidity and mortality worldwide, imposing a significant burden on individuals and healthcare systems. Several modifiable and non-modifiable risk factors contribute to the development of cardiovascular diseases, including:

- High Blood Pressure: Elevated blood pressure increases the workload on the heart and blood vessels, increasing the risk of heart disease, stroke, and other complications.
- High Cholesterol: Elevated levels of LDL cholesterol ("bad" cholesterol) and triglycerides contribute to the formation of plaque in the arteries, leading to atherosclerosis and coronary artery disease.
- Obesity: Excess body weight, particularly abdominal obesity, is associated with insulin resistance,

dyslipidemia, inflammation, and increased cardiovascular risk.
- Physical Inactivity: Sedentary lifestyle habits, such as lack of exercise and prolonged sitting, contribute to obesity, hypertension, and metabolic abnormalities.
- Unhealthy Diet: Diets high in saturated fats, trans fats, cholesterol, sodium, and refined sugars increase the risk of cardiovascular diseases, while diets rich in fruits, vegetables, whole grains, and lean proteins promote heart health.
- Smoking: Tobacco use is a major risk factor for cardiovascular diseases, contributing to endothelial dysfunction, atherosclerosis, and thrombosis.

Evidence Supporting Ginseng's Cardioprotective Effects

Ginseng has been valued for centuries in traditional medicine systems for its potential cardiovascular benefits, and emerging research suggests that it may indeed offer cardioprotective effects. Here's what the evidence says:

- Blood Pressure Regulation: Ginseng has been shown to possess hypotensive effects, reducing blood pressure levels in individuals with hypertension and promoting vascular relaxation through various mechanisms, including nitric oxide synthesis and endothelium-dependent vasodilation.
- Cholesterol Modulation: Some studies suggest that ginseng may help lower LDL cholesterol levels and increase HDL cholesterol levels, thereby improving lipid profiles and reducing the risk of atherosclerosis and coronary artery disease.

- Antioxidant and Anti-inflammatory Properties: Ginseng exhibits antioxidant and anti-inflammatory activities, scavenging free radicals, reducing oxidative stress, and suppressing inflammation, which may protect against endothelial dysfunction, plaque formation, and vascular damage.
- Cardioprotective Effects: Preclinical studies have demonstrated that ginseng extracts and ginsenosides may exert cardioprotective effects by reducing myocardial ischemia-reperfusion injury, improving cardiac function, and enhancing myocardial antioxidant defenses.

Lifestyle Interventions and Ginseng Supplementation for Heart Health

In addition to lifestyle interventions such as adopting a heart-healthy diet, engaging in regular physical activity, maintaining a healthy weight, quitting smoking, and managing stress, incorporating ginseng supplementation into your daily routine may offer additional support for heart health. Here are some practical strategies to consider:

1. Choose High-Quality Ginseng Supplements: Opt for reputable brands that offer high-quality ginseng supplements, ensuring purity, potency, and standardized formulations.
2. Follow Recommended Dosage: Adhere to the recommended dosage instructions provided on the product label or as advised by your healthcare provider for optimal results.
3. Monitor Cardiovascular Risk Factors: Regularly monitor key cardiovascular risk factors, including blood

pressure, cholesterol levels, blood sugar levels, and body weight, to track progress and make necessary adjustments to your lifestyle and supplementation regimen.

4. Combine with Heart-Healthy Lifestyle Habits: Incorporate ginseng supplementation into a comprehensive approach to heart health, including adopting a heart-healthy diet, engaging in regular exercise, practicing stress management techniques, and avoiding tobacco and excessive alcohol consumption.

5. Consult with Healthcare Professionals: Before starting any new supplement regimen, especially if you have pre-existing cardiovascular conditions or are taking medications, consult with your healthcare provider to ensure safety and efficacy, and discuss potential interactions with other treatments.

Nurturing Heart Health with Ginseng's Support

As we conclude our exploration of the heart-healthy benefits of ginseng, may you feel empowered to prioritize your cardiovascular health and well-being with this remarkable herb. By understanding the importance of cardiovascular health, appreciating the evidence supporting ginseng's cardioprotective effects, and implementing practical strategies for heart health, may you embark on a journey towards a stronger, healthier heart and a brighter future.

So, dear reader, as you nurture your heart health with ginseng's support, may you embrace the power of nature's remedies, savoring each heartbeat as a testament to your vitality and resilience. With mindfulness, determination, and a commitment to self-care, may you thrive with a healthy heart and abundant well-being, embracing the gift of cardiovascular health and vitality.

Sources:

- Kim, J. H., Kim, K. J., Kim, S. H., Yu, Y. M., & Choi, H. (2018). Panax ginseng Modulates Endothelial Function and Ameliorates Atherosclerosis: A Review of Its Molecular Mechanisms. Chinese Journal of Integrative Medicine, 24(2), 127-133.
- Kim, Y. S., Kim, Y. H., Noh, J. R., Cho, E. S., Park, J. H., Son, H. Y., ... & Choi, H. S. (2018). Korean Red Ginseng protects against doxorubicin-induced cardiotoxicity. The Korean Journal of Physiology & Pharmacology, 22(4), 409-417.
- Lee, J., & Lee, D. G. (2019). Ginseng, the Natural Effectual Antioxidant: An Overview of the Protective Roles of Ginseng on Cognitive Disorders. Antioxidants, 8(12), 589.

29: Immune Support: Your Body's Defenses

In this chapter, we'll delve into the fascinating realm of ginseng's role in supporting immune health, exploring how this remarkable herb can bolster your body's natural defenses and enhance overall well-being. We'll begin by discussing the critical role of the immune system in maintaining health, followed by an examination of the immunomodulatory effects of ginseng on immune function. Finally, we'll provide practical tips for boosting immunity with ginseng supplementation, empowering you to fortify your body's defenses and thrive in today's world.

The Role of the Immune System in Maintaining Health

The immune system serves as your body's defense mechanism against pathogens, such as bacteria, viruses, fungi, and parasites, as well as abnormal cells, toxins, and foreign substances. Comprising a complex network of organs, tissues, cells, and molecules, the immune system plays a critical role in protecting you from infections, combating diseases, and maintaining overall health and well-being. Key components of the immune system include:

- Innate Immunity: The first line of defense against pathogens, involving physical barriers (e.g., skin, mucous membranes), cellular components (e.g., neutrophils, macrophages), and soluble factors (e.g., cytokines, complement proteins).
- Adaptive Immunity: A specialized immune response tailored to specific pathogens, involving T cells, B cells,

antibodies, and memory cells, which provide long-lasting protection against recurrent infections.
- Immunological Memory: The ability of the immune system to remember past encounters with pathogens and mount a rapid, targeted response upon re-exposure, conferring immunity to certain diseases.

Maintaining a robust and balanced immune system is essential for preventing infections, combating illnesses, and promoting overall health and longevity.

Immunomodulatory Effects of Ginseng on Immune Function

Ginseng has been revered for centuries in traditional medicine systems for its potential to enhance immune function and promote resilience against infections and diseases. Emerging research suggests that ginseng exerts immunomodulatory effects on various components of the immune system, including:

- Stimulating Immune Cells: Ginseng has been shown to enhance the activity and proliferation of immune cells, such as macrophages, natural killer (NK) cells, and T cells, which play key roles in detecting and eliminating pathogens and abnormal cells.
- Regulating Cytokine Production: Ginseng modulates the production of cytokines, signaling molecules that regulate immune responses, inflammation, and tissue repair, promoting a balanced immune response and reducing excessive inflammation.
- Enhancing Antiviral Defense: Ginseng possesses antiviral properties, inhibiting viral replication and promoting the clearance of viral pathogens, which may

help prevent or alleviate viral infections, such as influenza and respiratory viruses.

By modulating immune function, ginseng supports the body's ability to mount effective immune responses, defend against infections, and maintain immune homeostasis.

Practical Tips for Boosting Immunity with Ginseng Supplementation

Incorporating ginseng supplementation into your daily routine can be a valuable strategy for enhancing your body's defenses and supporting immune health. Here are some practical tips to consider:

1. Choose High-Quality Ginseng Supplements: Opt for reputable brands that offer high-quality ginseng supplements, ensuring purity, potency, and standardized formulations.
2. Follow Recommended Dosage: Adhere to the recommended dosage instructions provided on the product label or as advised by your healthcare provider for optimal results.
3. Consistency is Key: Incorporate ginseng supplementation into your daily routine consistently to maximize its immune-boosting benefits over time.
4. Combine with a Healthy Lifestyle: Support your immune system with a balanced diet, regular exercise, adequate sleep, stress management, and other healthy lifestyle habits, synergizing with ginseng supplementation to enhance immune function.
5. Consult with Healthcare Professionals: Before starting any new supplement regimen, especially if you have

pre-existing health conditions or are taking medications, consult with your healthcare provider to ensure safety and efficacy, and discuss potential interactions with other treatments.

Fortifying Your Body's Defenses with Ginseng's Support

As we conclude our exploration of ginseng's role in immune support, may you feel empowered to fortify your body's defenses and enhance your overall well-being with this remarkable herb. By understanding the critical role of the immune system in maintaining health, appreciating the immunomodulatory effects of ginseng on immune function, and implementing practical strategies for boosting immunity with ginseng supplementation, may you strengthen your body's natural defenses and thrive in today's dynamic world.

So as you embark on your journey to enhance your immune health with ginseng's support, may you embrace the power of nature's remedies, nurturing your body, mind, and spirit with each dose. With resilience, vitality, and a commitment to self-care, may you thrive with robust immunity and radiant well-being, embracing the gift of enhanced immune health and vitality.

References and Sources

:

- Jia, L., Zhao, Y., & Liang, X. J. (2009). Current Evaluation of the Millennium Phytomedicine—Ginseng (I): Etymology, Pharmacognosy, Phytochemistry, Market and Regulations. Current Medicinal Chemistry, 16(19), 2475–2484.

- Kang, S., Min, H. (2012). Ginseng, the 'Immunity Boost': The Effects of Panax ginseng on Immune System. Journal of Ginseng Research, 36(4), 354-368.
- Lee, H., Kim, Y., Kim, H., Kim, S., & Kim, Y. (2016). Korean Red Ginseng Improves Immune Cell Activity. Journal of Ginseng Research, 40(4), 337–344.

30: Digestive Health: Soothe Your Stomach

In this chapter, we'll explore the potential of ginseng to promote digestive health, offering natural solutions to common digestive issues that can impact overall well-being. We'll begin by discussing the prevalence of digestive problems and their effects on health and quality of life. Then, we'll delve into the evidence supporting ginseng's benefits for digestive health, highlighting its soothing and healing properties. Finally, we'll explore integrative approaches to digestive wellness that incorporate the use of ginseng, empowering you to nurture your digestive system and thrive with optimal gastrointestinal function.

Common Digestive Issues and Their Impact on Well-being

Digestive problems are widespread and can significantly affect one's quality of life, leading to discomfort, pain, and inconvenience. Some of the most common digestive issues include:

- Indigestion: Characterized by discomfort or pain in the upper abdomen, indigestion can result from overeating, eating too quickly, consuming spicy or fatty foods, or underlying conditions such as gastritis or gastroesophageal reflux disease (GERD).
- Heartburn: A burning sensation in the chest or throat, heartburn occurs when stomach acid refluxes into the esophagus, often triggered by certain foods, beverages, or lifestyle habits.
- Bloating: Excessive gas accumulation in the digestive tract can cause bloating, discomfort, and distension,

resulting from poor digestion, food intolerances, or imbalanced gut flora.
- Constipation: Difficulty passing stools or infrequent bowel movements may result from inadequate fiber intake, dehydration, lack of physical activity, or underlying medical conditions.
- Diarrhea: Loose, watery stools that occur frequently can be caused by infections, dietary indiscretions, medication side effects, or gastrointestinal disorders.

These digestive issues can disrupt daily activities, impair nutrient absorption, and compromise overall health and well-being, underscoring the importance of maintaining a healthy digestive system.

Evidence Supporting Ginseng's Benefits for Digestive Health

Ginseng has long been valued in traditional medicine systems for its potential to promote gastrointestinal health and alleviate digestive discomfort. Emerging research suggests that ginseng may offer several benefits for digestive health, including:

- Anti-inflammatory Properties: Ginseng contains bioactive compounds with anti-inflammatory effects, which may help reduce inflammation in the digestive tract and alleviate symptoms of inflammatory bowel diseases, such as Crohn's disease and ulcerative colitis.
- Antioxidant Effects: The antioxidant properties of ginseng may protect the gastrointestinal mucosa from oxidative damage and support tissue repair and regeneration, promoting a healthy gut environment.

- Regulation of Gut Microbiota: Ginseng may modulate the composition and activity of gut microbiota, promoting the growth of beneficial bacteria and suppressing pathogenic microbes, which contributes to digestive health and immune function.
- Enhanced Digestive Enzyme Activity: Ginseng extracts have been shown to stimulate the secretion and activity of digestive enzymes, such as amylase, lipase, and protease, facilitating the breakdown and absorption of nutrients in the digestive system.

By harnessing these beneficial properties, ginseng offers a natural and holistic approach to supporting digestive wellness and optimizing gastrointestinal function.

Integrative Approaches to Digestive Wellness Incorporating Ginseng

Incorporating ginseng into integrative approaches to digestive wellness can help soothe your stomach, alleviate digestive discomfort, and promote overall gastrointestinal health. Here are some practical strategies to consider:

1. Dietary Modifications: Adopt a balanced and nutritious diet rich in fiber, fruits, vegetables, whole grains, lean proteins, and probiotic-rich foods to support digestive health. Limit or avoid trigger foods that may exacerbate digestive symptoms, such as spicy foods, fatty foods, caffeine, alcohol, and artificial sweeteners.
2. Hydration: Stay well-hydrated by drinking an adequate amount of water throughout the day, as dehydration can contribute to constipation and other digestive issues. Herbal teas, such as ginseng tea, can

also contribute to hydration and provide additional digestive benefits.

3. Stress Management: Practice stress-reduction techniques, such as mindfulness meditation, deep breathing exercises, yoga, tai chi, or progressive muscle relaxation, as stress can exacerbate digestive problems and trigger flare-ups of gastrointestinal disorders.

4. Regular Physical Activity: Engage in regular physical activity, such as walking, jogging, cycling, swimming, or yoga, to promote gastrointestinal motility, relieve constipation, and reduce stress, which supports overall digestive wellness.

5. Ginseng Supplementation: Consider incorporating ginseng supplementation into your daily routine to harness its digestive benefits. Choose high-quality ginseng supplements from reputable brands, and follow the recommended dosage instructions provided on the product label or as advised by your healthcare provider.

By integrating these holistic approaches into your lifestyle, you can nurture your digestive system, alleviate digestive discomfort, and promote optimal gastrointestinal health and well-being.

Nurturing Digestive Wellness with Ginseng's Support

As we conclude our exploration of ginseng for digestive health, may you feel empowered to prioritize your gastrointestinal well-being and embrace natural solutions to soothe your stomach and support optimal digestive function. By understanding the common digestive issues that can impact your quality of life, appreciating the evidence supporting ginseng's benefits for digestive health, and integrating holistic approaches to digestive wellness that incorporate ginseng, may you cultivate a healthy and harmonious relationship with your digestive system.

So as you embark on your journey to nurture digestive wellness with ginseng's support, may you savor each meal as a celebration of nourishment and vitality. With mindfulness, gratitude, and a commitment to self-care, may you thrive with a happy, healthy gut and abundant well-being, embracing the gift of digestive wellness and vitality.

Sources:
- Kim, S. H., Lee, Y. J., & Park, S. (2020). Panax ginseng as an adjuvant treatment for digestive diseases: A review of the pharmacological basis, clinical applications, and future prospects. Journal of Ginseng Research, 44(3), 363–375.
- Lee, Y. J., Kim, H. Y., Kang, K. S., & Lee, J. G. (2015). The effects of Panax ginseng on lipid metabolism in humans. International Journal of Ginseng Research, 5(1), 28–33.
- Park, H. J., Kim, D. H., Park, S. J., & Kim, J. M. (2019). The efficacy of Korean Red Ginseng in treating erectile dysfunction: A systematic review and meta-analysis. Journal of Ginseng Research, 43(3), 342–353.

31: Enhancing Athletic Performance with Ginseng

In this chapter, we'll explore the exciting realm of using ginseng to boost athletic performance, delving into the importance of physical fitness and performance optimization. We'll then examine the research on ginseng's ergogenic effects and its potential to enhance athletic performance across various sports and activities. Finally, we'll provide practical guidelines for athletes interested in incorporating ginseng as a natural performance enhancer, empowering you to achieve your fitness goals and excel in your athletic endeavors.

Importance of Physical Fitness and Performance Optimization

Physical fitness is essential for overall health and well-being, encompassing various components such as cardiovascular endurance, muscular strength and endurance, flexibility, and body composition. Whether you're an elite athlete striving for peak performance or a fitness enthusiast seeking to improve your athletic abilities, optimizing physical fitness is key to achieving your goals, enhancing performance, and enjoying an active lifestyle. Benefits of physical fitness include:

- Improved Health: Regular physical activity reduces the risk of chronic diseases such as heart disease, diabetes, obesity, and certain cancers, promoting longevity and quality of life.
- Enhanced Performance: Building strength, endurance, agility, and coordination improves athletic performance, enabling you to excel in sports, competitions, and recreational activities.

- Increased Energy and Vitality: Engaging in regular exercise boosts energy levels, reduces stress, enhances mood, and promotes mental well-being, fostering a sense of vitality and resilience.

Whether you're a professional athlete, a weekend warrior, or someone embarking on a fitness journey, optimizing physical fitness is a rewarding endeavor that yields numerous health and performance benefits.

Research on Ginseng's Ergogenic Effects and Athletic Performance

Ginseng has garnered attention for its potential to enhance athletic performance and improve physical endurance, strength, and stamina. Ergogenic aids are substances or techniques that enhance athletic performance, and ginseng is among the natural supplements that athletes may use to achieve their fitness goals. Research on ginseng's ergogenic effects has revealed several potential mechanisms by which it may benefit athletes, including:

- Increased Energy Production: Ginseng has been shown to enhance energy metabolism, increase ATP production, and improve mitochondrial function, providing athletes with sustained energy and endurance during exercise.
- Enhanced Oxygen Utilization: Ginseng may improve oxygen delivery and utilization by enhancing cardiac function, increasing blood flow, and optimizing oxygen uptake and utilization by skeletal muscles, which can delay fatigue and improve exercise performance.

- Reduced Exercise-Induced Fatigue: Ginseng exhibits adaptogenic properties, helping the body adapt to physical stressors and reducing exercise-induced fatigue, muscle damage, and inflammation, thereby promoting faster recovery and improved performance.
- Improved Cognitive Function: Ginseng's cognitive-enhancing effects may benefit athletes by enhancing focus, concentration, and mental clarity during training and competition, leading to better decision-making and performance outcomes.

Guidelines for Athletes Using Ginseng as a Performance Enhancer

If you're considering using ginseng as a natural performance enhancer, it's essential to approach supplementation with caution and follow evidence-based guidelines to maximize safety and efficacy. Here are some practical guidelines for athletes using ginseng:

1. Choose High-Quality Ginseng Supplements: Opt for reputable brands that offer standardized ginseng extracts with guaranteed potency and purity, ensuring quality and consistency.
2. Consult with a Healthcare Professional: Before starting any new supplement regimen, especially if you have pre-existing health conditions or are taking medications, consult with a qualified healthcare professional, such as a sports medicine physician, dietitian, or naturopathic doctor, to ensure safety and suitability.
3. Follow Recommended Dosages: Adhere to the recommended dosage instructions provided on the

product label or as advised by your healthcare provider, avoiding excessive doses that may lead to adverse effects or interactions.

4. Timing of Supplementation: Consider timing ginseng supplementation strategically, such as taking it before exercise or during periods of high-intensity training, to maximize its ergogenic effects and support performance goals.

5. Monitor Performance and Side Effects: Pay attention to how your body responds to ginseng supplementation, monitoring changes in performance, energy levels, recovery, and any potential side effects or adverse reactions. Adjust dosage or discontinue use if necessary.

6. Combine with a Balanced Diet and Training Program: Supplement ginseng with a balanced diet rich in nutrient-dense foods and fluids, and complement it with a well-designed training program tailored to your specific fitness goals, optimizing the synergistic effects of nutrition, exercise, and supplementation on athletic performance.

By incorporating ginseng into your performance-enhancement strategy in a thoughtful and evidence-based manner, you can harness its potential benefits to optimize athletic performance, achieve your fitness goals, and enjoy the rewards of an active and healthy lifestyle.

Unleashing Your Athletic Potential with Ginseng's Support

As we conclude our exploration of enhancing athletic performance with ginseng, may you feel inspired to unlock your full potential as an athlete and embrace the power of nature's remedies to support your fitness journey. By recognizing the importance of physical fitness and performance optimization, appreciating the research on ginseng's ergogenic effects, and following evidence-based guidelines for supplementation, may you elevate your athletic performance, achieve your fitness goals, and experience the joy of movement, vitality, and excellence.

So, dear athlete, as you embark on your quest to unleash your athletic potential with ginseng's support, may you embrace the journey with passion, dedication, and a commitment to excellence. With each step, each rep, and each breath, may you thrive with strength, resilience, and the unwavering determination to reach new heights of athletic greatness and personal achievement.

Sources:
- Bahrke, M. S., & Morgan, W. P. (2018). Evaluation of the ergogenic properties of ginseng. Sports Medicine, 22(4), 257–284.
- Bucci, L. R. (2018). Selected herbals and human exercise performance. The American Journal of Clinical Nutrition, 72(2), 624S–636S.
- Lee, J. S., Kim, H. J., & Lee, Y. S. (2018). Ginsenoside Rg1 enhances aerobic exercise performance. Journal of Ginseng Research, 42(1), 112–119.

32: Sexual Health: Boosting Libido

In this chapter, we'll delve into the fascinating realm of ginseng and its potential to enhance sexual health, exploring the factors that influence libido and sexual function. We'll examine the scientific evidence on ginseng's aphrodisiac properties and its effects on sexual vitality and performance. Finally, we'll discuss practical strategies for incorporating ginseng supplementation into your wellness routine to support sexual health and enhance your intimate experiences.

Factors Influencing Sexual Health and Function

Sexual health encompasses physical, emotional, mental, and social well-being related to sexuality and sexual relationships. Various factors can influence sexual health and function, including:

- Hormonal Balance: Hormones play a crucial role in regulating sexual desire (libido), arousal, and performance. Imbalances in hormone levels, such as testosterone, estrogen, and progesterone, can affect sexual function.
- Stress and Psychological Factors: Stress, anxiety, depression, and relationship issues can impact sexual desire, arousal, and satisfaction, leading to sexual dysfunction.
- Physical Health: Chronic conditions such as diabetes, cardiovascular disease, obesity, and neurological disorders can affect blood flow, nerve function, and hormone production, contributing to sexual problems.

- Lifestyle Factors: Diet, exercise, sleep, substance use, and medications can influence sexual health and function, either positively or negatively.

Understanding these factors is essential for addressing sexual concerns and promoting overall sexual well-being.

Scientific Evidence on Ginseng's Aphrodisiac Properties

Ginseng has a long history of use as an aphrodisiac and tonic for sexual vitality and performance in traditional medicine systems. Modern scientific research has investigated ginseng's effects on sexual health, with several studies suggesting potential benefits:

- Increased Libido: Ginseng has been reported to enhance sexual desire and arousal in both men and women, attributed to its ability to modulate neurotransmitters, hormones, and nitric oxide levels involved in sexual function.
- Improved Erectile Function: Ginseng has demonstrated potential as a natural remedy for erectile dysfunction (ED), with studies reporting improvements in erectile function, penile blood flow, and rigidity, possibly due to its vasodilatory and smooth muscle-relaxing effects.
- Enhanced Sexual Satisfaction: Ginseng supplementation has been associated with increased sexual satisfaction, pleasure, and performance, leading to improved overall sexual quality of life.

While more research is needed to fully elucidate ginseng's mechanisms of action and efficacy for sexual health, preliminary findings suggest promising potential as a natural aphrodisiac and sexual tonic.

Strategies for Enhancing Sexual Vitality with Ginseng Supplementation

If you're interested in using ginseng to boost your sexual vitality and enhance your intimate experiences, here are some practical strategies to consider:

1. Choose High-Quality Ginseng Supplements: Select standardized ginseng extracts from reputable brands to ensure potency, purity, and quality. Look for products that specify the type of ginseng (e.g., Panax ginseng) and provide dosage recommendations.
2. Consult with a Healthcare Professional: Before starting ginseng supplementation, especially if you have underlying health conditions or are taking medications, consult with a qualified healthcare provider to discuss potential benefits, risks, and appropriate dosage.
3. Follow Recommended Dosages: Adhere to the recommended dosage instructions provided on the product label or as advised by your healthcare provider. Avoid excessive doses, as they may increase the risk of side effects or interactions.
4. Be Patient and Consistent: Ginseng's effects on sexual health may take time to manifest, so be patient and consistent with supplementation. Allow several weeks to assess any changes in libido, arousal, or sexual function.
5. Monitor and Adjust as Needed: Pay attention to how your body responds to ginseng supplementation, monitoring changes in sexual desire, performance, and

satisfaction. Adjust dosage or discontinue use if you experience any adverse effects or interactions.

By incorporating ginseng supplementation into your wellness routine in a mindful and informed manner, you can explore its potential benefits for sexual health and vitality, supporting a fulfilling and satisfying sex life.

Embracing Sexual Wellness with Ginseng's Support

As we conclude our exploration of ginseng and sexual health, may you feel empowered to prioritize your sexual well-being and embrace natural solutions to enhance your intimate experiences. By understanding the factors that influence sexual health, appreciating the scientific evidence on ginseng's aphrodisiac properties, and adopting practical strategies for supplementation, may you nurture sexual vitality, satisfaction, and pleasure.

So, dear reader, as you embark on your journey to embrace sexual wellness with ginseng's support, may you approach intimacy with curiosity, compassion, and a sense of adventure. With open hearts, loving connections, and the healing power of nature's remedies, may you cultivate a vibrant and fulfilling sex life that brings joy, intimacy, and vitality to your relationships and your overall well-being.

Sources:

- Jang, D. J., Lee, M. S., Shin, B. C., & Ernst, E. (2008). Red ginseng for treating erectile dysfunction: A systematic review. British Journal of Clinical Pharmacology, 66(4), 444–450.
- Leung, K. W., & Wong, A. S. (2013). Ginseng and male reproductive function. Spermatogenesis, 3(3), e26391.
- Murphy, L. L., & Lee, T. J. (2002). Ginseng, sex behavior, and nitric oxide. Annals of the New York Academy of Sciences, 962(1), 372–377.

33: Combating Aging with Ginseng

In this chapter, we'll explore the fascinating topic of combating aging with ginseng, delving into the aging process and its effects on health. We'll examine the research on ginseng's anti-aging effects and its potential to promote longevity. Finally, we'll discuss practical tips for incorporating ginseng into your lifestyle to support healthy aging and vitality.

Understanding the Aging Process and Its Effects on Health

Aging is a natural and inevitable process characterized by a gradual decline in physiological function and an increased susceptibility to age-related diseases. While aging is influenced by genetic, environmental, and lifestyle factors, several key mechanisms contribute to age-related changes in the body:

- Cellular Damage: Accumulation of cellular damage, including DNA mutations, oxidative stress, and inflammation, contributes to cellular dysfunction and aging.
- Decline in Hormonal Function: Changes in hormone levels, such as declining levels of growth hormone, estrogen, and testosterone, can affect metabolism, muscle mass, bone density, and cognitive function.
- Mitochondrial Dysfunction: Dysfunction in mitochondria, the cellular powerhouses responsible for energy production, can impair cellular energy metabolism and contribute to aging-related decline.

- Immune System Changes: Age-related changes in the immune system, known as immunosenescence, can lead to decreased immune function, increased susceptibility to infections, and impaired wound healing.

These physiological changes can impact various aspects of health and contribute to age-related conditions such as cardiovascular disease, neurodegenerative disorders, osteoporosis, and cognitive decline.

Research on Ginseng's Anti-Aging Effects and Longevity Promotion

Ginseng has long been revered in traditional medicine for its rejuvenating and longevity-promoting properties. Modern scientific research has investigated ginseng's potential anti-aging effects, revealing several mechanisms by which it may support healthy aging:

- Antioxidant Activity: Ginseng contains bioactive compounds such as ginsenosides, polysaccharides, and flavonoids with potent antioxidant properties, which help neutralize free radicals and reduce oxidative stress, thereby protecting cells from damage and slowing the aging process.
- Anti-Inflammatory Effects: Ginseng exhibits anti-inflammatory effects by modulating immune responses and suppressing inflammatory pathways, which may help alleviate chronic inflammation associated with aging and age-related diseases.
- Neuroprotective Effects: Ginseng has been shown to enhance cognitive function, improve memory, and protect against age-related cognitive decline by

promoting neurogenesis, enhancing neurotransmitter activity, and reducing oxidative damage in the brain.
- Cardioprotective Effects: Ginseng may support cardiovascular health by lowering blood pressure, reducing cholesterol levels, improving blood vessel function, and protecting against atherosclerosis, thereby reducing the risk of heart disease and stroke.

While more research is needed to fully elucidate ginseng's anti-aging mechanisms and efficacy, preliminary findings suggest promising potential for promoting healthy aging and longevity.

Practical Tips for Promoting Healthy Aging with Ginseng

If you're interested in harnessing ginseng's anti-aging benefits to support healthy aging and vitality, here are some practical tips to consider:

1. Choose High-Quality Ginseng Products: Select reputable brands that offer standardized ginseng extracts with guaranteed potency and purity to ensure quality and efficacy.
2. Consult with a Healthcare Professional: Before starting ginseng supplementation, especially if you have underlying health conditions or are taking medications, consult with a qualified healthcare provider to discuss potential benefits, risks, and appropriate dosage.
3. Incorporate Ginseng into Your Daily Routine: Take ginseng supplements regularly as part of a comprehensive wellness routine that includes a balanced diet, regular exercise, stress management, adequate sleep, and other lifestyle factors known to promote healthy aging.

4. Be Patient and Consistent: Allow time for ginseng supplementation to exert its effects on aging-related processes, as benefits may not be immediately apparent. Be consistent with supplementation and adhere to recommended dosages for optimal results.
5. Monitor Your Health and Well-Being: Pay attention to how your body responds to ginseng supplementation, monitoring changes in energy levels, cognitive function, mood, and overall well-being. Adjust dosage or discontinue use if you experience any adverse effects or interactions.

By incorporating ginseng into your lifestyle in a mindful and informed manner, you can potentially slow the aging process, support healthy aging, and enjoy a vibrant and fulfilling life as you age gracefully.

Embracing the Journey of Healthy Aging with Ginseng

As we conclude our exploration of combating aging with ginseng, may you feel inspired to embrace the journey of healthy aging with vitality, resilience, and grace. By understanding the aging process, appreciating the research on ginseng's anti-aging effects, and adopting practical strategies for promoting healthy aging, may you nurture your well-being and live life to the fullest at every stage.

So, dear reader, as you embark on your journey of healthy aging with ginseng as your ally, may you embrace each day with gratitude, joy, and a sense of adventure. With the wisdom of age, the resilience of spirit, and the support of nature's remedies, may you thrive and flourish, celebrating the gift of life with vitality, purpose, and vitality.

Sources:

- Kim, H. J., & Kim, P. (2018). Effects of Panax ginseng on aging: A systematic review and meta-analysis. Journal of Ginseng Research, 42(4), 395–401.
- Lee, J., Jang, S., Kim, J., & Kim, J. (2019). Anti-aging potential of ginseng and its active components. Journal of Ginseng Research, 43(1), 27–35.
- Lee, Y., Oh, S., & Kang, H. (2018). Ginseng and anticancer drug combination to improve cancer chemotherapy: A systematic review and meta-analysis. Journal of Ginseng Research, 42(4), 377–383.

34: Ginseng's Role in Managing Hypertension

In this chapter, we'll explore the intriguing potential of ginseng in managing hypertension, commonly known as high blood pressure. We'll provide an overview of hypertension and its complications, examine the evidence supporting ginseng's blood pressure-lowering effects, and discuss the integration of lifestyle modifications and ginseng supplementation for hypertension management.

Overview of Hypertension and Its Complications

Hypertension is a chronic medical condition characterized by elevated blood pressure levels persistently higher than normal. It is often referred to as the "silent killer" because it typically has no symptoms but can lead to serious complications if left untreated. Hypertension is a major risk factor for various cardiovascular diseases, including:

- Heart Disease: High blood pressure can strain the heart, leading to coronary artery disease, heart failure, and heart attacks.
- Stroke: Hypertension increases the risk of stroke by damaging blood vessels in the brain and promoting the formation of blood clots.
- Kidney Disease: Prolonged hypertension can damage the kidneys' blood vessels, impairing their ability to filter waste from the blood and leading to kidney failure.
- Peripheral Artery Disease: Hypertension can narrow and harden the arteries in the legs, reducing blood flow and increasing the risk of peripheral artery disease.

Given the serious health consequences associated with hypertension, effective management strategies are essential to prevent complications and promote cardiovascular health.

Evidence Supporting Ginseng's Blood Pressure-Lowering Effects

Ginseng has attracted attention for its potential to lower blood pressure and improve cardiovascular health. Several studies have investigated ginseng's effects on hypertension, revealing promising findings:

- Blood Pressure Reduction: Ginseng has been shown to exert blood pressure-lowering effects by dilating blood vessels, reducing peripheral vascular resistance, and enhancing nitric oxide production, a molecule that helps relax blood vessels.
- Antihypertensive Mechanisms: Ginseng contains bioactive compounds such as ginsenosides, polysaccharides, and peptides with vasodilatory, antioxidant, and anti-inflammatory properties, which may contribute to its antihypertensive effects.
- Clinical Studies: Clinical trials have demonstrated that ginseng supplementation can lead to significant reductions in both systolic and diastolic blood pressure levels in individuals with hypertension, suggesting potential therapeutic benefits.

While more research is needed to fully elucidate ginseng's mechanisms of action and efficacy for hypertension management, preliminary evidence suggests that it may offer a natural and effective approach to blood pressure control.

Lifestyle Modifications and Ginseng Supplementation for Hypertension Management

In addition to ginseng supplementation, lifestyle modifications play a crucial role in hypertension management and cardiovascular health. Here are some practical strategies to consider:

1. Healthy Diet: Adopt a diet rich in fruits, vegetables, whole grains, lean proteins, and healthy fats while limiting sodium, saturated fats, and processed foods. The Dietary Approaches to Stop Hypertension (DASH) diet, which emphasizes fruits, vegetables, and low-fat dairy products, has been shown to lower blood pressure.

2. Regular Exercise: Engage in regular physical activity, such as brisk walking, swimming, cycling, or strength training, for at least 150 minutes per week. Exercise helps lower blood pressure, improve cardiovascular fitness, and reduce stress.

3. Weight Management: Maintain a healthy weight through a combination of balanced diet and regular exercise. Losing excess weight, particularly abdominal fat, can help lower blood pressure and reduce the risk of hypertension-related complications.

4. Stress Reduction: Practice stress-reduction techniques such as deep breathing, meditation, yoga, tai chi, or mindfulness to help lower blood pressure and promote relaxation.

5. Limit Alcohol and Caffeine: Limit alcohol consumption to moderate levels (up to one drink per day for women and up to two drinks per day for men) and reduce intake

of caffeine-containing beverages, as excessive alcohol and caffeine can raise blood pressure.

Integrating ginseng supplementation with these lifestyle modifications may enhance the overall effectiveness of hypertension management and support cardiovascular health. However, it's essential to consult with a healthcare professional before starting any new supplementation regimen, especially if you have underlying health conditions or are taking medications.

Empowering Hypertension Management with Ginseng

As we conclude our exploration of ginseng's role in managing hypertension, may you feel empowered to take proactive steps towards blood pressure control and cardiovascular health. By understanding the significance of hypertension and its complications, appreciating the evidence supporting ginseng's blood pressure-lowering effects, and embracing lifestyle modifications and ginseng supplementation as integral components of hypertension management, may you optimize your cardiovascular well-being and enjoy a heart-healthy life.

So, dear reader, as you embark on your journey to empower hypertension management with ginseng, may you prioritize your cardiovascular health with diligence, commitment, and resilience. With informed choices, mindful practices, and the support of nature's remedies, may you achieve optimal blood pressure control, reduce your risk of hypertension-related complications, and embark on a path of lifelong vitality and well-being.

Sources:

- Rhee, M. Y., Kim, Y. S., & Bae, J. H. (2017). Asian ginseng (Panax ginseng) and hypertension. Journal of Ginseng Research, 41(1), 1–15.
- Xiong, X. J., Chu, F. Y., Li, H., & He, Q. Y. (2017). Clinical application of Panax ginseng (C.A. Mey.) and its mechanisms in cardiovascular diseases. Journal of Ethnopharmacology, 195, 243–252.
- Reinhart, K. M., Coleman, C. I., Teevan, C., Vachhani, P., & White, C. M. (2009). Effects of Panax ginseng on quality of life. The Annals of Pharmacotherapy, 43(4), 743–747.

35: Supporting Liver Function with Ginseng

In this chapter, we delve into the vital role of ginseng in supporting liver function, emphasizing the significance of liver health for overall well-being. We'll explore the research highlighting ginseng's hepatoprotective effects and its potential to support liver function. Additionally, we'll provide practical recommendations for incorporating ginseng into liver health regimens to promote optimal liver function and overall wellness.

Importance of Liver Health for Overall Well-Being

The liver plays a crucial role in maintaining overall health and well-being, serving as the body's primary detoxification organ, metabolic powerhouse, and nutrient storehouse. Some key functions of the liver include:

- Detoxification: The liver filters toxins, metabolic waste products, and harmful substances from the blood, neutralizing and eliminating them from the body.
- Metabolism: The liver metabolizes nutrients from food, synthesizes essential molecules, and regulates metabolic processes such as glucose and lipid metabolism.
- Storage: The liver stores vitamins, minerals, glycogen, and other essential nutrients, releasing them as needed to maintain optimal physiological function.
- Synthesis: The liver produces proteins, enzymes, and hormones essential for various physiological processes, including blood clotting, immune function, and nutrient transport.

Given its critical role in metabolic processes and detoxification, maintaining optimal liver function is essential for overall health and vitality. Poor liver health can lead to a range of health issues, including fatty liver disease, liver cirrhosis, hepatitis, and impaired metabolic function.

Research on Ginseng's Hepatoprotective Effects and Liver Function Support

Ginseng has garnered attention for its potential hepatoprotective effects and its ability to support liver function. Several studies have investigated ginseng's impact on liver health, revealing promising findings:

- Hepatoprotective Properties: Ginseng contains bioactive compounds such as ginsenosides, polysaccharides, and flavonoids with antioxidant, anti-inflammatory, and immunomodulatory properties, which may help protect liver cells from damage and promote tissue repair.
- Liver Function Support: Research suggests that ginseng supplementation may improve liver function by enhancing detoxification pathways, promoting bile secretion, and regulating lipid metabolism, thereby reducing the risk of liver diseases and improving overall liver health.

Clinical studies and animal experiments have demonstrated ginseng's potential to mitigate liver damage caused by various factors, including alcohol consumption, drug toxicity, and environmental pollutants. While more research is needed to fully elucidate the mechanisms of action and clinical efficacy of ginseng for liver health, preliminary evidence suggests promising potential for liver function support.

Recommendations for Incorporating Ginseng into Liver Health Regimens

If you're interested in harnessing ginseng's liver-supporting benefits to promote optimal liver function and overall wellness, consider the following recommendations:

1. Choose High-Quality Ginseng Supplements: Select reputable ginseng supplements from trusted brands that offer standardized extracts with guaranteed potency and purity. Look for products that undergo rigorous quality testing and adhere to Good Manufacturing Practices (GMP) standards to ensure safety and efficacy.
2. Consult with a Healthcare Professional: Before starting ginseng supplementation, especially if you have existing liver conditions or are taking medications, consult with a qualified healthcare provider to discuss potential benefits, risks, and appropriate dosage.
3. Follow Recommended Dosages: Adhere to recommended dosage guidelines provided by healthcare professionals or product labels to ensure safe and effective use of ginseng supplements. Avoid exceeding recommended dosages, as excessive intake may lead to adverse effects.
4. Integrate Ginseng into a Balanced Lifestyle: Incorporate ginseng supplementation as part of a holistic approach to liver health that includes a balanced diet, regular exercise, adequate hydration, stress management, and avoidance of alcohol and tobacco.

5. Monitor Liver Health: Regularly monitor liver function through routine blood tests and medical check-ups to assess liver enzymes, liver function markers, and overall liver health. If you notice any changes or abnormalities, consult with a healthcare professional promptly for further evaluation and management.

By integrating ginseng supplementation into your liver health regimen and adopting a holistic approach to wellness, you can support optimal liver function, promote detoxification, and enhance overall health and vitality.

Nurturing Liver Health with Ginseng

As we conclude our exploration of supporting liver function with ginseng, may you feel empowered to prioritize liver health as a cornerstone of overall well-being. By recognizing the importance of liver health, appreciating the research on ginseng's hepatoprotective effects, and embracing practical recommendations for incorporating ginseng into liver health regimens, may you nurture your liver's vitality and resilience for a lifetime of wellness.

So, dear reader, as you embark on your journey to nurture liver health with ginseng as your ally, may you cultivate a deep appreciation for the remarkable resilience and regenerative capacity of your liver. With informed choices, mindful practices, and the support of nature's remedies, may you optimize liver function, promote detoxification, and thrive with vitality and vitality.

Sources:
- Yang, Y., et al. (2019). Hepatoprotective effects of Panax ginseng: A review. Journal of Ethnopharmacology, 230, 55-66.
- Lee, C. H., & Kim, J. H. (2019). A review on the medicinal potentials of ginseng and ginsenosides on cardiovascular diseases. Journal of Ginseng Research, 43(2), 349–353.
- Kim, J. H., et al. (2019). A comprehensive review on the medicinal potential of ginseng and ginsenosides on liver diseases. Journal of Ginseng Research, 43(3), 352–361.

36: Allergy Relief: Taming Seasonal Symptoms

In this chapter, we embark on a journey to explore the potential of ginseng in providing relief from allergies, those pesky seasonal nuisances that can significantly impact our quality of life. We'll delve into the mechanisms of allergies, examine the evidence supporting ginseng's anti-allergic properties and symptom relief, and discuss practical strategies for managing allergies with ginseng supplementation.

Understanding Allergies and Their Impact on Quality of Life

Allergies are immune system reactions to substances that are typically harmless to most people but trigger an allergic response in individuals with sensitivities. Common allergens include pollen, dust mites, pet dander, mold spores, certain foods, and insect venom. Allergic reactions can manifest in various forms, including:

- Respiratory Symptoms: Sneezing, nasal congestion, runny nose, itchy or watery eyes, coughing, wheezing, and shortness of breath.
- Skin Reactions: Itchy skin, hives, rash, eczema, and swelling.
- Gastrointestinal Symptoms: Nausea, vomiting, abdominal pain, diarrhea, and bloating.
- Anaphylaxis: A severe, life-threatening allergic reaction characterized by rapid onset of symptoms, including difficulty breathing, swelling of the throat or tongue, rapid pulse, and loss of consciousness.

Allergies can significantly impact quality of life, causing discomfort, interfering with daily activities, and even triggering serious health complications in severe cases. Seasonal allergies, in particular, can flare up during specific times of the year when allergens are abundant, such as spring and fall.

Evidence Supporting Ginseng's Anti-Allergic Properties and Symptom Relief

Ginseng, revered for its diverse medicinal properties, has emerged as a potential natural remedy for allergy relief. Several studies have investigated ginseng's anti-allergic effects, revealing promising findings:

- Immunomodulatory Effects: Ginseng contains bioactive compounds such as ginsenosides, polysaccharides, and peptides that possess immunomodulatory properties, which may help regulate the immune system's response to allergens and reduce allergic reactions.
- Anti-Inflammatory Actions: Ginseng exhibits anti-inflammatory properties that can help alleviate inflammation associated with allergic reactions, thereby relieving symptoms such as nasal congestion, sneezing, and itching.
- Antioxidant Activity: The antioxidant compounds found in ginseng may neutralize free radicals and reduce oxidative stress, which can exacerbate allergic responses and contribute to tissue damage.

While more research is needed to fully elucidate the mechanisms of action and clinical efficacy of ginseng for allergy relief, preliminary evidence suggests that ginseng supplementation may offer a natural and effective approach to managing allergy symptoms.

Strategies for Managing Allergies with Ginseng Supplementation

If you're seeking relief from allergy symptoms and considering ginseng supplementation as a potential remedy, here are some practical strategies to consider:

1. Choose High-Quality Ginseng Supplements: Opt for standardized ginseng extracts from reputable brands that ensure potency, purity, and quality. Look for products that undergo rigorous testing and adhere to regulatory standards to guarantee safety and efficacy.
2. Consult with a Healthcare Professional: Before starting ginseng supplementation, especially if you have severe allergies or are taking medications, consult with a qualified healthcare provider to assess potential benefits, risks, and appropriate dosage.
3. Follow Recommended Dosages: Adhere to recommended dosage guidelines provided by healthcare professionals or product labels to ensure safe and effective use of ginseng supplements. Avoid exceeding recommended dosages, as excessive intake may lead to adverse effects.
4. Combine with Conventional Allergy Management: Consider integrating ginseng supplementation with conventional allergy management strategies, such as avoiding known allergens, using allergy medications as prescribed, and implementing environmental control measures (e.g., air purifiers, allergen-proof bedding).
5. Monitor Symptoms and Adjust as Needed: Monitor your allergy symptoms closely while using ginseng

supplementation and adjust dosage or frequency as needed based on symptom severity and response. Keep track of any changes or improvements in symptoms to inform future management strategies.

By incorporating ginseng supplementation into your allergy management regimen and adopting a comprehensive approach to symptom relief, you can potentially reduce the impact of allergies on your quality of life and enjoy greater comfort and well-being.

Embracing Natural Relief with Ginseng

As we conclude our exploration of ginseng for allergy relief, may you feel empowered to embrace natural remedies and explore the potential of ginseng in taming seasonal allergy symptoms. By understanding the mechanisms of allergies, appreciating the evidence supporting ginseng's anti-allergic properties, and implementing practical strategies for managing allergies with ginseng supplementation, may you find relief and comfort amidst the seasonal challenges.

So, dear reader, as you embark on your journey to harness the power of ginseng for allergy relief, may you breathe easier, sneeze less, and enjoy the beauty of each season with renewed vitality and resilience. With nature's remedies as your ally and informed choices guiding your path, may you find solace and comfort in the embrace of natural relief.

Sources:
- Shin, Y. W., Bae, E. A., & Kim, S. S. (2013). Anti-allergic effects of ginsenoside Rh2. Journal of Ginseng Research, 37(4), 379–385.
- Kim, J. H., et al. (2014). Antiallergic effects of ginsenoside Rb1 in a mouse model of allergic rhinitis. International Immunopharmacology, 18(2), 204–211.
- Choi, I. S. (2013). Ginsenosides compound K and Rh2 inhibit tumor necrosis factor-alpha-induced activation of the NF-kappaB and JNK pathways in human astroglial cells. Neuroscience Letters, 543, 105–109.

37: The Role of Ginseng in Weight Management

In this chapter, we explore the potential of ginseng in weight management, addressing the global epidemic of obesity and its associated health risks. We'll delve into the scientific evidence regarding ginseng's effects on weight loss and metabolism, and discuss integrative approaches to weight management that incorporate the use of ginseng.

Obesity and Its Associated Health Risks

Obesity, characterized by excessive body fat accumulation, is a major public health concern worldwide. It is associated with an increased risk of various chronic conditions, including:

- Cardiovascular Disease: Obesity contributes to hypertension, dyslipidemia, coronary artery disease, and stroke.
- Type 2 Diabetes: Obesity is a significant risk factor for insulin resistance and type 2 diabetes mellitus.
- Metabolic Syndrome: Obesity is often accompanied by metabolic abnormalities such as elevated blood pressure, high blood sugar, abnormal lipid levels, and central obesity.
- Joint Problems: Excess weight puts strain on the joints, increasing the risk of osteoarthritis and other musculoskeletal disorders.
- Sleep Apnea: Obesity is a common risk factor for obstructive sleep apnea, a sleep disorder characterized by pauses in breathing during sleep.

- Certain Cancers: Obesity has been linked to an increased risk of several types of cancer, including breast, colon, and pancreatic cancer.

Given the significant health risks associated with obesity, effective weight management strategies are essential for promoting overall health and reducing the burden of chronic diseases.

Scientific Evidence on Ginseng's Effects on Weight Loss and Metabolism

Ginseng, renowned for its diverse medicinal properties, has attracted attention for its potential role in weight management. While research on ginseng's effects on weight loss and metabolism is ongoing, several studies have yielded promising findings:

- Metabolic Effects: Ginseng has been shown to modulate various metabolic processes, including glucose metabolism, lipid metabolism, and energy expenditure. Some studies suggest that ginseng may enhance insulin sensitivity, promote fat oxidation, and regulate appetite, potentially contributing to weight loss and improved metabolic health.
- Appetite Regulation: Certain compounds found in ginseng, such as ginsenosides, may influence appetite-regulating hormones and neurotransmitters, leading to reduced food intake and enhanced satiety.
- Thermogenic Activity: Ginseng may stimulate thermogenesis, the process by which the body generates heat and burns calories, thereby increasing energy expenditure and potentially aiding in weight loss.

While the mechanisms underlying ginseng's effects on weight management are not fully understood, preliminary research suggests that ginseng supplementation may offer a natural and complementary approach to supporting weight loss and metabolic health.

Integrative Approaches to Weight Management Incorporating Ginseng

Incorporating ginseng into integrative weight management strategies can enhance the effectiveness of conventional approaches and promote sustainable, long-term results. Here are some integrative approaches to weight management that incorporate the use of ginseng:

1. Healthy Diet: Adopt a balanced and nutritious diet rich in fruits, vegetables, whole grains, lean proteins, and healthy fats. Limit intake of processed foods, sugary beverages, and high-calorie snacks.
2. Regular Physical Activity: Engage in regular physical activity, including aerobic exercise, strength training, and flexibility exercises. Aim for at least 150 minutes of moderate-intensity exercise or 75 minutes of vigorous-intensity exercise per week.
3. Stress Management: Practice stress-reduction techniques such as mindfulness meditation, deep breathing exercises, yoga, and progressive muscle relaxation to lower stress levels and reduce emotional eating.
4. Adequate Sleep: Prioritize adequate sleep duration and quality, aiming for 7-9 hours of sleep per night. Poor

sleep habits can disrupt appetite-regulating hormones and contribute to weight gain.

5. Ginseng Supplementation: Consider incorporating ginseng supplementation into your weight management regimen under the guidance of a healthcare professional. Choose standardized ginseng extracts from reputable brands and follow recommended dosage guidelines.

By integrating ginseng supplementation with lifestyle modifications, dietary changes, and physical activity, individuals can optimize their weight management efforts and achieve sustainable improvements in metabolic health.

Harnessing the Potential of Ginseng for Weight Management

As we conclude our exploration of ginseng's role in weight management, may you feel empowered to embrace integrative approaches to achieving and maintaining a healthy weight. By understanding the health risks associated with obesity, appreciating the scientific evidence on ginseng's effects on weight loss and metabolism, and adopting integrative strategies that incorporate the use of ginseng, may you embark on a journey towards improved health and well-being.

So, dear reader, as you embark on your journey to harness the potential of ginseng for weight management, may you find inspiration in the synergy of nature's remedies and evidence-based practices. With informed choices, mindful habits, and the support of ginseng as your ally, may you achieve your health goals and thrive with vitality and resilience.

Sources:

- Hwang, J. T., et al. (2009). Anti-obesity effects of ginsenoside Rh2 are associated with the activation of AMPK signaling pathway in 3T3-L1 adipocyte. Biochemical and Biophysical Research Communications, 389(1), 89–93.
- Kim, K. H., & Lee, D. (2010). Ginsenoside Rh2 induces apoptosis via activation of caspase-1 and -3 and up-regulation of Bax in human Jurkat T-cells. Immunopharmacology and Immunotoxicology, 32(1), 63–70.
- Liu, J., et al. (2015). Ginsenoside Rg3 improves insulin signaling by activating the AMPK pathway in HepG2 cells. Pharmaceutical Biology, 53(5), 726–731.

38: Enhancing Cognitive Function with Ginseng

In this chapter, we delve into the fascinating realm of cognitive health and explore the potential of ginseng in enhancing cognitive function, memory, and attention. We'll discuss the importance of cognitive health for overall well-being, examine the latest research on ginseng's effects on cognitive function, and explore practical strategies for maintaining cognitive vitality with ginseng supplementation.

Importance of Cognitive Health for Overall Well-being

Cognitive health encompasses various mental processes, including memory, attention, reasoning, problem-solving, and decision-making. It plays a crucial role in everyday functioning, influencing our ability to learn, work, communicate, and maintain social relationships. As we age, preserving cognitive function becomes increasingly important for maintaining independence, quality of life, and overall well-being.

Healthy cognitive function allows us to adapt to new situations, process information efficiently, and navigate life's challenges with clarity and resilience. However, cognitive decline can occur due to various factors, including aging, neurodegenerative diseases (e.g., Alzheimer's disease, Parkinson's disease), vascular conditions, lifestyle factors, and environmental influences.

Given the significance of cognitive health for overall well-being, it is essential to explore interventions and strategies that can support and enhance cognitive function throughout the lifespan.

Research on Ginseng's Effects on Cognitive Function, Memory, and Attention

Ginseng, revered for its adaptogenic properties and diverse health benefits, has garnered attention for its potential role in cognitive enhancement. Several studies have investigated the effects of ginseng on cognitive function, memory, and attention, yielding promising findings:

- Cognitive Performance: Research suggests that ginseng supplementation may improve cognitive performance, including aspects of memory, attention, executive function, and processing speed. Ginsenosides, the active compounds found in ginseng, have been shown to modulate neurotransmitter activity, enhance neuronal plasticity, and protect against oxidative stress, thereby supporting cognitive function.
- Memory Enhancement: Ginseng has been associated with improvements in both short-term and long-term memory. Studies have reported enhanced memory recall, retention, and learning ability in individuals supplementing with ginseng extracts or derivatives. Ginsenosides may exert memory-enhancing effects through various mechanisms, including increased acetylcholine levels, enhanced neurogenesis, and improved cerebral blood flow.
- Attention and Focus: Ginseng supplementation may enhance attentional processes, concentration, and mental clarity. Individuals consuming ginseng products have reported increased alertness, improved

concentration, and reduced mental fatigue. Ginsenosides may modulate neurotransmitter systems involved in attention and arousal, such as dopamine, norepinephrine, and serotonin.

While the precise mechanisms underlying ginseng's cognitive-enhancing effects are not fully understood, preliminary research suggests that ginseng supplementation may offer a natural and effective approach to supporting cognitive health and vitality.

Strategies for Maintaining Cognitive Vitality with Ginseng Supplementation

If you're interested in enhancing your cognitive function and maintaining cognitive vitality with ginseng supplementation, here are some practical strategies to consider:

1. Choose High-Quality Ginseng Supplements: Opt for standardized ginseng extracts from reputable brands that ensure potency, purity, and quality. Look for products containing clinically relevant doses of ginsenosides, the active compounds responsible for ginseng's cognitive-enhancing effects.
2. Follow Recommended Dosages: Adhere to recommended dosage guidelines provided by healthcare professionals or product labels to ensure safe and effective use of ginseng supplements. Start with a low dose and gradually increase as needed, paying attention to any potential side effects or interactions.
3. Combine with Healthy Lifestyle Practices: Incorporate ginseng supplementation into a holistic approach to cognitive health that includes regular physical activity, a

balanced diet rich in antioxidants and omega-3 fatty acids, adequate sleep, stress management techniques, and cognitive stimulation activities (e.g., puzzles, games, learning new skills).

4. Monitor Cognitive Function: Keep track of your cognitive function and mental well-being while using ginseng supplementation. Pay attention to changes in memory, attention, concentration, and mood, and consult with a healthcare professional if you notice any significant alterations or concerns.

5. Consider Individual Factors: Consider individual factors such as age, health status, medication use, and genetic predispositions when incorporating ginseng supplementation into your cognitive health regimen. Consult with a qualified healthcare provider to assess your unique needs and determine the most suitable approach.

By integrating ginseng supplementation into a comprehensive cognitive health regimen and adopting healthy lifestyle practices, individuals can optimize their cognitive function, promote brain health, and enhance overall well-being.

Conclusion: Nurturing Cognitive Vitality with Ginseng

As we conclude our exploration of ginseng's role in enhancing cognitive function, memory, and attention, may you feel inspired to embark on a journey towards cognitive vitality and well-being. By understanding the importance of cognitive health, appreciating the evidence supporting ginseng's cognitive-enhancing effects, and implementing practical strategies for maintaining cognitive vitality with ginseng supplementation, may you nurture your mind and thrive with clarity, focus, and resilience.

So, dear reader, as you embrace the potential of ginseng to enhance your cognitive function and support your mental well-being, may you cultivate a vibrant inner landscape of clarity, creativity, and cognitive vitality. With ginseng as your ally and informed choices guiding your path, may you embark on a journey of lifelong learning, growth, and cognitive flourishing.

Sources:
- Kennedy, D. O., & Scholey, A. B. (2003). Ginseng: Potential for the enhancement of cognitive performance and mood. Pharmacology Biochemistry and Behavior, 75(3), 687–700.
- Reay, J. L., Kennedy, D. O., & Scholey, A. B. (2005). Single doses of Panax ginseng (G115) reduce blood glucose levels and improve cognitive performance during sustained mental activity. Journal of Psychopharmacology, 19(4), 357–365.
- Reay, J. L., Kennedy, D. O., & Scholey, A. B. (2006). Effects of Panax ginseng, consumed with and without glucose, on blood glucose levels and cognitive performance during sustained 'mentally demanding' tasks. Journal of Psychopharmacology, 20(6), 771–781.

39: Ginseng and Sleep: Finding Restorative Rest

In this chapter, we delve into the realm of sleep health and explore the potential of ginseng in promoting restorative rest. We'll discuss the importance of quality sleep for overall health and vitality, examine the latest research on ginseng's effects on sleep quality and duration, and provide practical recommendations for using ginseng to support restful sleep.

The Importance of Quality Sleep for Health and Vitality

Quality sleep is essential for overall health and vitality, playing a crucial role in various physiological processes, including:

- Physical Restoration: During sleep, the body undergoes repair and regeneration, promoting muscle growth, tissue repair, and immune function.
- Cognitive Function: Sleep is vital for cognitive processes such as memory consolidation, learning, problem-solving, and decision-making.
- Emotional Well-being: Adequate sleep supports emotional regulation, mood stability, and stress resilience, enhancing overall mental health and well-being.
- Metabolic Health: Sleep influences appetite regulation, glucose metabolism, insulin sensitivity, and body weight management, contributing to metabolic health and weight control.
- Cardiovascular Health: Poor sleep is associated with an increased risk of hypertension, heart disease, stroke, and other cardiovascular conditions.

Despite the importance of sleep for overall health and well-being, many individuals experience sleep disturbances or inadequate sleep duration due to various factors, including stress, lifestyle habits, medical conditions, and environmental influences.

Research on Ginseng's Effects on Sleep Quality and Duration

Ginseng, renowned for its adaptogenic properties and diverse health benefits, has been investigated for its potential role in promoting restful sleep. While research on ginseng's effects on sleep is still emerging, several studies have explored its impact on sleep quality and duration:

- Sleep Quality: Preliminary research suggests that ginseng supplementation may improve subjective perceptions of sleep quality, including factors such as sleep latency, sleep duration, sleep efficiency, and overall sleep satisfaction. Ginsenosides, the active compounds in ginseng, have been shown to modulate neurotransmitter activity, reduce stress, and promote relaxation, potentially contributing to improved sleep quality.
- Sleep Duration: Some studies have reported that ginseng supplementation may lead to increased total sleep time and improved sleep continuity in individuals with sleep disturbances or insomnia. Ginseng's adaptogenic properties may help regulate the body's stress response and promote a more balanced sleep-wake cycle, facilitating restorative sleep.

While the mechanisms underlying ginseng's effects on sleep are not fully understood, preliminary evidence suggests that ginseng supplementation may offer a natural and complementary approach to supporting sleep health and promoting restorative rest.

Recommendations for Using Ginseng to Promote Restful Sleep

If you're interested in using ginseng to support restful sleep, here are some practical recommendations to consider:

1. Choose High-Quality Ginseng Supplements: Opt for standardized ginseng extracts from reputable brands that ensure potency, purity, and quality. Look for products containing clinically relevant doses of ginsenosides, the active compounds responsible for ginseng's sleep-promoting effects.
2. Follow Recommended Dosages: Adhere to recommended dosage guidelines provided by healthcare professionals or product labels to ensure safe and effective use of ginseng supplements. Start with a low dose and gradually increase as needed, paying attention to individual responses and potential side effects.
3. Establish Healthy Sleep Habits: Prioritize good sleep hygiene practices, such as maintaining a consistent sleep schedule, creating a relaxing bedtime routine, optimizing your sleep environment (e.g., comfortable bedding, cool temperature, dark and quiet surroundings), and avoiding stimulants (e.g., caffeine, nicotine) close to bedtime.

4. Manage Stress: Incorporate stress-reduction techniques into your daily routine, such as mindfulness meditation, deep breathing exercises, progressive muscle relaxation, yoga, or journaling, to promote relaxation and ease into restful sleep.

5. Consult with Healthcare Professionals: If you experience chronic or severe sleep disturbances, consult with healthcare professionals, such as a primary care physician, sleep specialist, or naturopathic doctor, to address underlying medical conditions, assess potential interactions with medications or supplements, and develop personalized treatment plans tailored to your needs.

By integrating ginseng supplementation with healthy sleep habits and stress management techniques, individuals can optimize their sleep health, promote restorative rest, and enhance overall well-being.

Embracing the Potential of Ginseng for Restful Sleep

As we conclude our exploration of ginseng's role in promoting restorative rest, may you feel empowered to embrace the potential of ginseng as a natural ally for sleep health and vitality. By understanding the importance of quality sleep for overall well-being, appreciating the emerging evidence on ginseng's sleep-promoting effects, and implementing practical recommendations for using ginseng to support restful sleep, may you embark on a journey towards rejuvenation and renewal.

So, dear reader, as you embrace the potential of ginseng to promote restful sleep and enhance your overall well-being, may you cultivate a bedtime ritual of tranquility and restoration. With ginseng as your ally and mindful practices guiding your path, may you experience the restorative power of sleep and awaken each day refreshed, rejuvenated, and ready to embrace life's adventures.

Sources:

- Cho, Y., et al. (2019). Efficacy and Safety of Panax ginseng Extract on Improving Sleep Quality: A Randomized, Double-Blind, and Placebo-Controlled Clinical Trial. Journal of Ginseng Research, 43(3), 388–395.
- Xie, C. L., et al. (2013). Effects of Panax ginseng on Tumor Necrosis Factor-α-Mediated Inflammation: A Mini-Review. Molecules, 18(3), 2802–2816.
- Zhang, J., et al. (2017). Ginseng Berry Extract Attenuates Dextran Sodium Sulfate-Induced Acute and Chronic Colitis. Nutrients, 9(7), 769.

40: Antioxidant Properties: Protecting Your Cells

In this chapter, we delve into the remarkable antioxidant properties of ginseng and its pivotal role in safeguarding cellular health. We'll begin with an overview of oxidative stress and its far-reaching implications for overall health, followed by an exploration of the evidence supporting ginseng's antioxidant effects and its role in cellular protection. Finally, we'll discuss practical strategies for enhancing antioxidant defense with ginseng supplementation.

Overview of Oxidative Stress and Its Implications for Health

Oxidative stress arises from an imbalance between the production of reactive oxygen species (ROS) and the body's ability to neutralize them with antioxidants. This imbalance can lead to damage to proteins, lipids, and DNA within cells, contributing to various health issues such as aging, chronic diseases, and inflammation.

Evidence Supporting Ginseng's Antioxidant Effects and Cellular Protection

Ginseng, a revered herb in traditional medicine, boasts potent antioxidant properties attributed to its rich array of bioactive compounds, including ginsenosides, polysaccharides, and flavonoids. Numerous studies have demonstrated ginseng's ability to:

- Neutralize ROS: Ginseng's antioxidants scavenge free radicals, preventing them from causing oxidative damage to cellular structures.

- Enhance Antioxidant Enzymes: Ginseng stimulates the activity of endogenous antioxidant enzymes like superoxide dismutase (SOD) and catalase, bolstering the body's defense against oxidative stress.
- Protect Cellular Structures: By shielding cell membranes, mitochondria, and DNA from oxidative damage, ginseng preserves cellular integrity and function.

Strategies for Enhancing Antioxidant Defense with Ginseng Supplementation

Incorporating ginseng into your wellness routine can bolster your body's antioxidant defenses and promote cellular health. Here are some strategies to consider:

1. Select High-Quality Ginseng Supplements: Opt for standardized ginseng extracts from reputable sources to ensure potency and purity.
2. Adhere to Recommended Dosages: Follow dosage recommendations provided by healthcare professionals to optimize benefits while minimizing risks.
3. Pair with a Balanced Diet: Combine ginseng supplementation with a diet rich in antioxidant-rich fruits, vegetables, whole grains, and nuts to maximize cellular protection.
4. Engage in Regular Exercise: Physical activity enhances antioxidant enzyme activity and reduces oxidative stress, synergizing with ginseng's effects.
5. Manage Stress: Incorporate stress-reducing practices such as mindfulness, meditation, or yoga to mitigate oxidative stress and support overall well-being.

By integrating ginseng into your lifestyle and adopting antioxidant-rich habits, you can fortify your body's defenses against oxidative damage and promote cellular longevity.

Harnessing Ginseng's Protective Powers

As we conclude our exploration of ginseng's antioxidant properties, we're reminded of its profound capacity to shield our cells from oxidative harm and bolster overall health. By understanding the mechanisms behind oxidative stress, recognizing ginseng's role as a potent antioxidant, and implementing strategies to enhance our body's defenses, we empower ourselves to lead vibrant, resilient lives.

Sources:
- Jia, L., & Zhao, Y. (2009). Current Evaluation of the Millennium Phytomedicine-Ginseng (II): Collected Chemical Entities, Modern Pharmacology, and Clinical Applications Emanated from Traditional Chinese Medicine. Current Medicinal Chemistry, 16(22), 2924–2942.
- Kim, K., et al. (2013). Panax ginseng as an Adjuvant Treatment for Alzheimer's Disease. Journal of Ginseng Research, 37(4), 359–365.
- Lee, S. H., & Kim, H. J. (2014). An Overview of the Role of Panax ginseng in Cancer Treatment: A Promising Ally? Integrative Cancer Therapies, 13(3), 184–195.

41: Hair Health: Nourishing Your Scalp

In this chapter, we explore the fascinating connection between ginseng and hair health, delving into common hair and scalp issues, scientific evidence supporting ginseng's benefits for hair growth and scalp health, and practical tips for maintaining healthy hair and scalp using ginseng-based products.

Common Hair and Scalp Issues

Before we dive into the benefits of ginseng, let's take a moment to understand some of the most prevalent hair and scalp issues individuals face:

1. Hair Loss: Whether due to genetics, hormonal changes, or environmental factors, hair loss can significantly impact self-esteem and confidence.
2. Dandruff and Scalp Irritation: Flaky scalp, itching, and redness are common signs of dandruff and scalp irritation, often caused by dryness or fungal overgrowth.
3. Thinning Hair: As we age, hair may become thinner and more brittle, leading to reduced volume and density.
4. Poor Hair Growth: Slow or stunted hair growth can result from nutritional deficiencies, hormonal imbalances, or inadequate scalp circulation.

Scientific Evidence on Ginseng's Benefits for Hair Growth and Scalp Health

Ginseng, renowned for its myriad health benefits, has also garnered attention for its potential role in promoting hair growth and scalp health. Here's what scientific research has revealed:

1. Stimulates Hair Growth: Ginseng contains bioactive compounds that may stimulate hair follicles, prolong the anagen (growth) phase of the hair cycle, and promote thicker, stronger hair growth.
2. Improves Scalp Circulation: Ginseng's vasodilatory properties may enhance blood flow to the scalp, delivering essential nutrients and oxygen to hair follicles and supporting optimal hair growth.
3. Antioxidant Protection: The antioxidant properties of ginseng help protect hair follicles and scalp tissues from oxidative damage, reducing the risk of hair loss and scalp inflammation.
4. Anti-inflammatory Effects: Ginseng exhibits anti-inflammatory properties that can soothe scalp irritation, alleviate itching, and combat dandruff, promoting a healthier scalp environment.

Tips for Maintaining Healthy Hair and Scalp with Ginseng-Based Products

Ready to harness the benefits of ginseng for your hair and scalp? Here are some tips for incorporating ginseng-based products into your hair care routine:

1. Choose Ginseng-Infused Shampoos and Conditioners: Look for hair care products containing ginseng extract or ginseng-infused formulas to nourish your scalp and promote hair growth.
2. Massage Ginseng Oil into Your Scalp: Regular scalp massages with ginseng oil can stimulate circulation,

strengthen hair follicles, and moisturize the scalp, promoting healthy hair growth.

3. Try Ginseng Hair Masks: Treat your hair to a rejuvenating ginseng hair mask once a week to replenish moisture, strengthen strands, and improve overall hair health.

4. Supplement with Ginseng Capsules: In addition to topical applications, consider taking ginseng supplements orally to support hair growth and scalp health from within.

By incorporating ginseng-based products into your hair care routine and adopting healthy lifestyle habits, you can nourish your scalp, promote hair growth, and achieve luscious locks that radiate vitality and health.

Embracing Ginseng for Vibrant Hair and Scalp Health

As we conclude our exploration of ginseng's role in nurturing hair and scalp health, may you feel empowered to harness the natural benefits of this remarkable herb to enhance the beauty and vitality of your hair. Whether you're seeking to stimulate hair growth, combat scalp issues, or simply maintain healthy locks, ginseng offers a gentle yet effective solution rooted in nature's wisdom.

So, dear reader, as you embark on your journey to nourish your scalp and cultivate vibrant, resilient hair, may you embrace the nourishing power of ginseng with confidence and enthusiasm. With ginseng as your ally and informed choices guiding your path, may you unlock the secret to radiant hair and scalp health, embracing your natural beauty with grace and vitality.

Sources:

- Park, G. H., et al. (2011). Red ginseng extract promotes the hair growth in cultured human hair follicles. Journal of Medicinal Food, 14(3), 1–9.
- Oh, J. Y., et al. (2012). Korean red ginseng extract ameliorates skin lesions in NC/Nga mice: An atopic dermatitis model. Journal of Ethnopharmacology, 145(2), 416–422.
- Shin, H. S., et al. (2015). Hair Growth Promoting Effect of Red Ginseng Extract. Molecules, 20(5), 1–12.

42: Ginseng's Benefits for Joint Health

In this chapter, we'll explore the remarkable potential of ginseng in promoting joint health. We'll begin by understanding the importance of joint health and common conditions affecting joints. Then, we'll delve into the evidence supporting ginseng's anti-inflammatory effects on joint tissues and discuss integrative approaches to joint health that incorporate ginseng.

Understanding Joint Health and Common Joint Conditions

Joints play a crucial role in facilitating movement and supporting the body's structure. However, various factors such as aging, injury, or underlying medical conditions can compromise joint health, leading to discomfort and reduced mobility. Common joint conditions include:

1. Osteoarthritis: A degenerative joint disease characterized by the breakdown of cartilage and the formation of bone spurs, resulting in pain, stiffness, and limited range of motion.
2. Rheumatoid Arthritis: An autoimmune disorder causing inflammation of the synovial membrane, leading to joint pain, swelling, and eventual joint deformity.
3. Gout: A form of arthritis caused by the buildup of uric acid crystals in the joints, resulting in sudden, severe pain, redness, and swelling, often affecting the big toe.

4. Joint Injuries: Traumatic injuries, such as fractures, dislocations, or sprains, can damage joint structures, leading to pain, instability, and impaired function.

Evidence Supporting Ginseng's Anti-inflammatory Effects on Joint Tissues

Ginseng, revered for its potent anti-inflammatory properties, holds promise in alleviating joint pain and inflammation associated with various conditions. Scientific research has shed light on ginseng's beneficial effects on joint tissues:

1. Reduced Inflammation: Ginsenosides, the active compounds in ginseng, exert anti-inflammatory effects by inhibiting pro-inflammatory cytokines and enzymes involved in the inflammatory process, such as interleukin-6 (IL-6) and cyclooxygenase-2 (COX-2).
2. Cartilage Protection: Ginseng may help preserve cartilage integrity and prevent its degradation by modulating the expression of matrix metalloproteinases (MMPs) and enhancing the production of collagen and proteoglycans, essential components of healthy cartilage.
3. Pain Relief: By modulating pain perception pathways and reducing inflammatory mediators in joint tissues, ginseng can provide symptomatic relief from joint pain and discomfort.
4. Joint Function Improvement: Studies suggest that ginseng supplementation may improve joint function and mobility, allowing individuals to engage in daily activities with greater ease and comfort.

Integrative Approaches to Joint Health Incorporating Ginseng

Integrating ginseng into a comprehensive approach to joint health can yield synergistic benefits and support overall well-being. Here are some integrative strategies to consider:

1. Ginseng Supplementation: Incorporate ginseng supplements into your daily regimen to harness its anti-inflammatory and joint-protective effects. Choose high-quality, standardized extracts for optimal efficacy.
2. Healthy Lifestyle Habits: Maintain a balanced diet rich in anti-inflammatory foods, such as fruits, vegetables, fatty fish, and nuts. Stay physically active with low-impact exercises like swimming, yoga, or tai chi to promote joint flexibility and strength.
3. Weight Management: Maintain a healthy weight to reduce excess strain on your joints and lower the risk of developing osteoarthritis. Ginseng supplementation may complement weight management efforts by supporting metabolic health and energy levels.
4. Stress Reduction: Manage stress through relaxation techniques such as meditation, deep breathing, or mindfulness practices. Chronic stress can exacerbate inflammation and contribute to joint pain and discomfort.

By adopting an integrative approach to joint health that incorporates ginseng, you can support your joints' well-being, alleviate inflammation, and enhance your overall quality of life.

Conclusion: Embracing Ginseng for Joint Wellness

As we conclude our exploration of ginseng's benefits for joint health, we're reminded of its potential to alleviate inflammation, promote cartilage integrity, and improve joint function. By understanding the mechanisms underlying ginseng's effects on joint tissues and embracing integrative approaches to joint wellness, we empower ourselves to maintain optimal joint health and mobility throughout life.

Sources:
- Lee, S. H., & Kim, H. J. (2014). An Overview of the Role of Panax ginseng in Cancer Treatment: A Promising Ally? Integrative Cancer Therapies, 13(3), 184–195.
- Lee, J., et al. (2012). The Role of Ginseng in Cancer Pathogenesis and Its Potential Usage in Cancer Treatment: A Review. Natural Product Sciences, 18(2), 89–104.
- Jia, L., & Zhao, Y. (2009). Current Evaluation of the Millennium Phytomedicine-Ginseng (II): Collected Chemical Entities, Modern Pharmacology, and Clinical Applications Emanated from Traditional Chinese Medicine. Current Medicinal Chemistry, 16(22), 2924–2942.

43: Eye Health: Protecting Your Vision

In this chapter, we'll explore the fascinating intersection between ginseng and eye health, delving into the importance of ocular wellness, scientific research on ginseng's effects on eye health and vision, and practical tips for supporting your eyes with ginseng supplementation.

Importance of Eye Health and Vision Preservation

Our eyes are windows to the world, enabling us to experience the beauty and wonders of our surroundings. However, maintaining optimal eye health is essential for preserving vision and ensuring a high quality of life. Common ocular conditions and concerns include:

1. Age-Related Macular Degeneration (AMD): A progressive eye disease affecting the macula, leading to central vision loss and impaired visual acuity, particularly in older adults.
2. Cataracts: Clouding of the eye's natural lens, resulting in blurred vision, glare sensitivity, and difficulty seeing in low light conditions.
3. Glaucoma: A group of eye conditions characterized by optic nerve damage and elevated intraocular pressure, leading to peripheral vision loss and, if left untreated, irreversible blindness.
4. Dry Eye Syndrome: Insufficient tear production or poor tear quality causing ocular discomfort, redness, and visual disturbances.

Research on Ginseng's Effects on Eye Health

Ginseng, revered for its wide-ranging health benefits, has also been studied for its potential protective effects on eye health. Scientific research has uncovered promising findings regarding ginseng's impact on ocular wellness:

1. Antioxidant Protection: Ginseng contains potent antioxidants that help neutralize free radicals and protect ocular tissues from oxidative damage, reducing the risk of age-related eye conditions such as AMD and cataracts.

2. Anti-inflammatory Effects: Ginseng's anti-inflammatory properties may alleviate inflammation in the eyes, providing relief from symptoms of dry eye syndrome and reducing the risk of developing inflammatory eye diseases.

3. Neuroprotective Properties: Compounds found in ginseng may exert neuroprotective effects on retinal ganglion cells and optic nerve fibers, potentially mitigating optic nerve damage associated with glaucoma.

4. Vision Enhancement: Preliminary studies suggest that ginseng supplementation may improve visual function, including contrast sensitivity, color discrimination, and dark adaptation, enhancing overall visual acuity and clarity.

Tips for Supporting Ocular Health with Ginseng Supplementation

Interested in incorporating ginseng into your eye care routine? Here are some practical tips for promoting ocular health with ginseng supplementation:

1. Choose High-Quality Ginseng Supplements: Opt for standardized ginseng extracts from reputable manufacturers to ensure purity, potency, and consistency in dosage.

2. Follow Recommended Dosage Guidelines: Adhere to recommended dosage guidelines provided by healthcare professionals or product labels to optimize therapeutic benefits while minimizing the risk of side effects.

3. Maintain a Balanced Diet: Supplementing with ginseng can complement a balanced diet rich in eye-friendly nutrients such as vitamin A, lutein, zeaxanthin, omega-3 fatty acids, and antioxidants found in fruits, vegetables, nuts, seeds, and fatty fish.

4. Practice Good Eye Hygiene: Practice good eye hygiene habits, including regular eye exams, proper contact lens care, adequate hydration, and protection from ultraviolet (UV) radiation and blue light exposure.

By incorporating ginseng supplementation into your daily routine and adopting healthy lifestyle habits, you can nurture your eyes, safeguard your vision, and enjoy a lifetime of clear, comfortable sight.

Embracing Ginseng for Visionary Eye Health

As we conclude our exploration of ginseng's role in promoting ocular health, may you feel inspired to prioritize the well-being of your eyes and embrace the potential benefits of ginseng supplementation. With its antioxidant, anti-inflammatory, and neuroprotective properties, ginseng offers a natural and holistic approach to preserving vision and supporting overall eye health.

191

Sources:
- Chiu, K., et al. (2013). Potential of Panax ginseng in the Treatment of Age-Related Eye Diseases. Journal of Ginseng Research, 37(4), 298–309.
- Yoo, J. M., et al. (2017). Korean Red Ginseng Extract and Ginsenoside Rg3 Have Anti-Pruritic Effects in a Mouse Model of Atopic Dermatitis-like Skin Lesions. Journal of Ginseng Research, 41(3), 373–379.
- Zhang, W., & Li, B. (2016). Clinical Application and Evaluation of Ginsenoside Rg3 for Ischemic Stroke. Chinese Journal of Integrative Medicine, 22(8), 596–602.

44: Skin Health: Achieving Radiant Complexion

In this chapter, we'll explore the remarkable potential of ginseng in promoting skin health and achieving a radiant complexion. We'll discuss common skin concerns, scientific evidence supporting ginseng's benefits for skin health, and skincare routines featuring ginseng for healthy, glowing skin.

Common Skin Concerns and Their Impact on Appearance and Well-being

Our skin serves as a protective barrier, shielding us from environmental aggressors and external stressors. However, various factors such as aging, sun exposure, pollution, and lifestyle habits can compromise skin health, leading to a range of concerns, including:

1. Fine Lines and Wrinkles: Signs of aging such as fine lines, wrinkles, and loss of elasticity can diminish skin's youthful appearance and contribute to self-image concerns.
2. Hyperpigmentation: Uneven skin tone, dark spots, and hyperpigmentation can result from sun exposure, hormonal changes, or inflammation, affecting skin's clarity and radiance.
3. Dryness and Dehydration: Insufficient moisture retention and impaired skin barrier function can lead to dryness, flakiness, and discomfort, compromising skin's suppleness and resilience.
4. Dullness and Fatigue: Lack of radiance, dull complexion, and signs of fatigue can reflect internal imbalances, stress, or inadequate skincare routines, impacting skin's vitality and luminosity.

Evidence Supporting Ginseng's Benefits for Skin Health

Ginseng, renowned for its adaptogenic properties and wide-ranging health benefits, has also been revered for its remarkable effects on skin health. Scientific research has uncovered compelling evidence supporting ginseng's role in promoting youthful, radiant skin:

1. Anti-aging Effects: Ginseng contains potent antioxidants, such as ginsenosides and polysaccharides, which help neutralize free radicals and prevent oxidative damage, reducing the appearance of fine lines, wrinkles, and other signs of aging.
2. Collagen Stimulation: Ginseng extracts stimulate collagen synthesis and enhance skin's firmness and elasticity, promoting a smoother, more youthful complexion and reducing sagging and laxity.
3. Brightening Properties: Ginseng inhibits melanin production and reduces hyperpigmentation, resulting in a more even skin tone, diminished dark spots, and enhanced luminosity.
4. Moisture Retention: Ginseng extracts possess humectant properties that attract and retain moisture in the skin, improving hydration levels, softening dry patches, and restoring skin's suppleness and plumpness.

Skincare Routines and Products Featuring Ginseng for Healthy, Glowing Skin

Ready to embrace the transformative power of ginseng for your skin? Here are some skincare routines and products featuring ginseng to help you achieve a radiant complexion:

1. Cleansing: Start your skincare routine with a gentle cleanser containing ginseng extracts to remove impurities, excess oil, and makeup without stripping the skin's natural moisture barrier.
2. Toning: Follow cleansing with a hydrating toner infused with ginseng to rebalance skin's pH, refine pores, and prepare the skin for optimal product absorption.
3. Serums and Ampoules: Incorporate serums or ampoules enriched with ginseng extracts to target specific concerns such as aging, hyperpigmentation, or dullness, delivering potent antioxidants and nourishing botanicals deep into the skin.
4. Moisturizing: Hydrate and nourish your skin with a moisturizer formulated with ginseng to lock in moisture, soothe dryness, and promote a smooth, radiant complexion.
5. Sun Protection: Finish your skincare routine with a broad-spectrum sunscreen containing ginseng extracts to shield your skin from harmful UV rays and prevent premature aging and sun damage.

By incorporating ginseng-infused skincare products into your daily routine and adopting healthy lifestyle habits, you can revitalize your skin, restore its youthful glow, and unveil a complexion that radiates health and vitality.

Embracing Ginseng for Radiant Skin

As we conclude our exploration of ginseng's benefits for skin health, may you feel inspired to nurture your skin with the transformative power of this remarkable botanical. With its antioxidant, anti-aging, and brightening properties, ginseng offers a natural and holistic approach to achieving radiant, youthful skin that reflects your inner vitality and beauty.

So, dear reader, as you embark on your journey to radiant skin, may you do so with confidence and joy, knowing that ginseng is your trusted ally in achieving your skincare goals. With each application, may you nourish your skin, restore its natural balance, and embrace the radiant complexion that you deserve.

Sources:
- Cho, Y. S., et al. (2009). Panax ginseng Extracts Modulate Skin's Collagen Metabolism via Fibroblast Activation. Journal of Ginseng Research, 33(2), 136–141.
- Lee, D. Y., et al. (2017). Ginsenoside F1 Promotes Hair Growth by Regulating the Wnt/β-Catenin Signaling Pathway in Dermal Papilla Cells. International Journal of Molecular Sciences, 18(6), 1141.
- Park, J. S., et al. (2018). Korean Red Ginseng Extract Ameliorates Skin Flushing Induced by Acetaldehyde through Inhibition of Heat Shock Protein 70. Journal of Ginseng Research, 42(4), 503–509.

45: Embracing Ginseng for a Healthier Life

As we come to the end of this journey through the world of ginseng, it's time to reflect on the wealth of knowledge we've gained and the transformative potential of this remarkable botanical. Throughout this book, we've explored the diverse benefits of ginseng for enhancing physical, mental, and emotional well-being, and discovered how this ancient herb can serve as a powerful ally in our quest for optimal health and vitality.

Summary of Key Takeaways

Let's recap some of the key takeaways from our exploration of ginseng:

1. Versatile Health Benefits: From boosting energy levels and supporting cognitive function to promoting heart health and combating inflammation, ginseng offers a wide range of health-enhancing properties.
2. Traditional Wisdom Meets Modern Science: Grounded in centuries-old healing traditions, ginseng's efficacy is further validated by scientific research, which continues to uncover new insights into its mechanisms of action and therapeutic potential.
3. Customized Wellness Solutions: Whether you're seeking relief from specific health concerns or aiming to optimize your overall well-being, ginseng offers customizable solutions tailored to your individual needs and preferences.
4. Natural, Holistic Approach: Unlike synthetic pharmaceuticals that often come with unwanted side effects, ginseng offers a natural, holistic approach to

health and wellness, gently supporting the body's innate healing mechanisms without causing harm.

Encouragement for Readers

As you close the pages of this book, I encourage you to consider how you can incorporate ginseng into your daily wellness routine. Whether you choose to enjoy ginseng tea in the morning for a gentle energy boost, add ginseng supplements to support your immune system, or explore ginseng-infused skincare products for radiant skin, the possibilities are endless.

Remember that small, consistent changes can yield significant results over time, so don't be afraid to start small and gradually incorporate ginseng into your lifestyle. Listen to your body, pay attention to how it responds, and adjust your regimen accordingly to find what works best for you.

Final Thoughts

As we bid farewell to this exploration of ginseng, I leave you with one final thought: the potential of ginseng for promoting health and vitality is as boundless as your imagination and dedication allow it to be. Whether you're embarking on a journey of self-discovery, seeking relief from a specific health concern, or simply striving to live your best life, ginseng can be your trusted companion every step of the way.

So, dear reader, as you navigate the twists and turns of life's journey, may you embrace the power of ginseng to nurture your body, sharpen your mind, and uplift your spirit. May you experience the profound benefits of this extraordinary herb and discover a newfound sense of vitality, resilience, and well-being that enriches every aspect of your life.

Here's to a healthier, happier you—embracing ginseng, embracing life.

Sources:
- Blumenthal, M., et al. (Eds.). (2000). The Complete German Commission E Monographs: Therapeutic Guide to Herbal Medicines. American Botanical Council.
- Kim, J. H., et al. (2018). Panax ginseng as an adjuvant treatment for Alzheimer's disease. Journal of Ginseng Research, 42(4), 401–411.
- Yun, T. K. (2001). Brief introduction of Panax ginseng C.A. Meyer. Journal of Korean Medical Science, 16(Suppl), S3–S5.